# WISDOM FROM
# CANCER CAREGIVERS JOURNEY

## LESSONS LEARNED

## RICHARD E. FARMER

Wisdom From Cancer Caregivers Journey:  Lessons Learned
ISBN 979-8-9861485-0-2  Softbound
ISBN 979-8-9861485-1-9  Hardbound

Request for information should be addressed to:
Curry Brothers Marketing and Publishing Group
P.O. Box 247 Haymarket, VA 20168

Executive Editing by Candace Curry-Williams
Cover Design and Graphics by Vibranium Media Group
Manuscript Formatting Vibranium Media Group

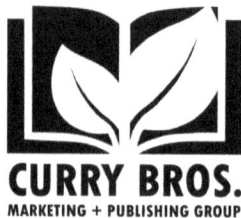

**CURRY BROS.**
MARKETING + PUBLISHING GROUP

# WISDOM FROM
# CANCER
# CAREGIVERS
# JOURNEY
## LESSONS LEARNED

### RICHARD E. FARMER

# Wisdom From Cancer Caregivers Journey: Lessons Learned

# Table of Contents

**Website**

www.cancertravelers.com

# Special Dedication

This book is dedicated to Dr. David W. Persky for his intensive efforts in helping with the development of this book.

In all instances including discussion of topics, selection of participant authors, and editing work for each author's contribution in the 5 Chapters of the book, Dr. Persky assumed a leadership role to help in all of the stages of this publication. Without any hesitancy, David participated in this publication through his volunteer work in virtually every aspect of the book from conceptual to actual aspects. He readily assumed a role of helper-facilitator as we brought the book from the initial concept stage to actual publication.

# The Journey of Cancer Giving
# By
# Richard E. Farmer

To start the conversation about the effects of cancer upon the caregivers, a poem/prayer seems to be necessary for setting the right tone for the pages which are presented. The following "mantra" was developed by Dr. Bonnie C. Farmer in 2015 and is modeled after the work of Jack Kornfield's Meditation on Loving Kindness (https://jackkornfield.com/meditation-loving_kindness/. So, this is written by Bonnie Cashin Farmer (2015)

My Loving Kindness Mantra

Please say or repeat….

May you be well
May you be happy
May you have peace
May you be free
May you not suffer
May you be loved
May God grant you mercy and divine intervention

Follow with inserting names of…...

Yourself
Your Spouse
Your Family

Then……

Others, perhaps someone you know or know of who appears to need help, extra blessings, or caring thoughts

Some neutral person or stranger, someone who slammed a door in your face, or inappropriately pulled out of an intersection and almost hit your car while paying no attention. Lastly, someone that you know or know of, whom you dislike or, someone who has wronged you, someone whose very name repels you.

Bonnie reports that she tries to practice loving kindness every day. Practicing Loving Kindness on a regular basis has the power to open your heart and reinforce the good in the world. Please keep in mind that there is no right way to practice, just do whatever manner of practice meets your needs.

# The Art and Science of Caregiving: Love

There is little doubt that caregiving is both an art and a science. For the most part, more than 90% or more of caregivers in the United States are spouses or other family members. Daily, they provide services to their cancer patients on a 24-hour basis. This requires that the new caregiver rapidly acquire the skills necessary to provide general medical care, drug distribution, food, and other forms of nutrition, plus general hygiene care as needed. Also, the comfort of the cancer patient must be attended to in terms of bedding, clothing, and movement equipment such as walkers, wheelchairs, canes, and the like. Transportation to the many medical providers is also required. Entertainment such as television and books for reading need also be the responsibility of the caregiver.

Ultimately, caregiving involves providing the physical, psychological, and emotional elements which are at the heart of love, and which is the basis of marriage and familial relationships. These then become the foundation and definition of what we know as caregiving. In the end, it is love for each other that provides the very basis of the care provided to cancer patients. In the end, we provide the care that we do because we love the patient. And, with love at hand, we are able to understand the individual with cancer which allows us to exercise compassion for that person. And true compassion is nothing more than a heartfelt form of love for the other albeit cancer diseased person.

Love is often associated with the concept of intimacy. For most, intimate knowledge of the other often produces change in ourselves. This change in effect puts us in an emotional cage. This experience contains both positive and negative thoughts and ideas. The cage creates positivity and negativity in our thinking and behavior. Curiously, positivity seems to be on a type of emotional timer which has both a turn on and turn off emotional component while negativity has no timer in the cage. It is clearly up to us to turn the negativity off so that we are not locked into a set of thoughts and ideas that have difficulties or problems associated with it. In the very end, it is singularly up to us to take control of these thoughts and feelings that are fundamentally negative. And this process of control of thoughts is also known as coping.

So, where does one go from here?

First, incorporating the idea that intimacy changes over time must be recognized by all caregivers. And because of this recognition, there is a need for perspectives that will help us to embrace this change. There is a need for a model of thinking called the Stress Behavior Model. This helps us to integrate the Stress Behavior Model to fight negative issues such as Post Traumatic Stress Disorder (PTSD).

Second, with PTSD as a model for understanding, what happens to all of us when we are suddenly confronted with the knowledge that our loved one has contracted cancer? This suddenly terrifying situation can result in any number of reactions such as vivid flashbacks to a more relaxing and peaceful situations, intrusive thoughts or images, nightmares, intense distress at prior experiences with you and the cancer patient, and physical sensations at the mere thought of prior highly pleasant situations with you and the cancer patient.

Third, the PTSD reactions or other reactions can be best delt with by incorporating stress behavioral principles into your thinking about your loved one suddenly conflicted with cancer. The stress-behavior model was conceived as a method to understand what we do when confronted with things like the PTSD behaviors. This is a process that includes recognition of the "stressors" we experience when we think about the cancer altering your relationship with the patient. This involves recognizing and identifying the "source" of the feeling, and the effects that this has upon us both physically and emotionally. Next comes the "effects" of the sources upon us both physically, emotionally, and socially. Finally, the coping behaviors that we employ to cope with the sources and its effects upon us.

You are encouraged to create a paper form which on the left side of the paper you write the words in a column, source, effects, and behaviors leaving ample space in the column for the three words. These should cover the entire length of the paper. In the middle of the paper form, you provide a wide column to record you effects or feelings of what the source does to you either physically or psychologically. Finally, the remaining space on the paper is for behaviors that you engage in when you experience the source and effects. In the end, this will give you a tool that will assist you in being a better caregiver for your patient. So, you are encouraged to go ahead and experiment with the form even to having multiple pages of the form to cover a whole series of sources.

As one military scholar reported that they, the military, are trained to respond and not react. The idea here is that we need to "train" ourselves so that we can respond and not just react. The Stress-Behavior Model thinking is a great way to begin the process of training ourselves so that we can respond to the needs of the cancer patient, and not just react to their requests or your determination of their needs at a given moment. The idea here is that merely reacting to a situation will often not give us the best response to a caregiving situation. Rather, training ourselves to respond is by far a better form to being a good caregiver then by simply reacting "from the gut" to a caregiving situation.

This book is the result of the experiences of 6 individuals as they have coped with being a caregiver to a cancer patient, commonly a spouse or other family member. There are five common themes or topics that each author has written. These themes have been developed by Richard E. Farmer as a result of his experience coping with his cancer diagnosis and the effect that this has had upon his life. He was diagnosed with Multiple Myeloma Cancer in the Fall of 2014. While there is at present no known cure for this cancer, Richard is in a close state of remission due to the successful treatment of chemotherapy. The themes that are presented here are reflections on personal experiences with cancer, essays, vignettes, and short stories designed to illustrate the theme. These have been developed by Richard fully based on his own experiences as a cancer patient learning to live a new and different life based upon his diagnosis.

It is vitally important for us to use the stress-behavior process to best understand what is going on with both the cancer patient and ourselves as caregivers. By knowing what is happening with both, we are in a better position to develop more healthy or less destructive behaviors. The idea here is that the more we know about the patient and ourselves, the better off we are as we attempt to construct coping behaviors which are healthy or less destructive to both the patient and the caregiver.

## Book Themes

The themes that are presented here are Being a Cancer Patient, Obtaining Support, Hope, Saying Goodbye, and Living a Meaningful Life. A final theme which is called Lessons Learned will synthesize the five experiences as briefly described by the author's themselves and summarized by the last author, David W. Persky.

## Being a Cancer Patient

This section will provide an overview of the cancer journey starting at the pre-diagnosis stage and ending at the conclusion of treatment and/or chemotherapy. This could focus briefly on how the cancer started, diagnosed; followed by including your feelings, attitudes, and so forth associated with this new status of life.

## Obtaining Support

Reflections in this section might would include your views, attitudes, needs for support. A description of what support looks like to you and how it feels when addressing how we can call on others to help us coping with our cancer. Can our support be identified when experienced? This could involve how we have reached out or not to caregivers, co-workers, fellow patients, and providers to help us better develop an understanding of our new status as a cancer patient from a healthful point-of-view. Does the meaning of support change over time and how? A cancer patient who has lived with uncurable cancer for six years could likely experience a change in how support is viewed. An interesting reflection might be how has support changed throughout the course of treatments, setbacks, decline, and recovery from acute medical-cancer events. And the concept of support also raises the issue of how we can reciprocate to the other members of our support group.

## Hope
Hope is a critical attitude for the maintenance of positive mental health in all people and is especially critically important for the cancer patient. Possessing hope gives us the ability to purposely direct our lives in a positive direction. And hope helps us to produce a balance between living in the present and some living directed toward the future. Reflections on hope might include, for example, what do you hope for? Do the goals of your hope change over time with disease management and or disease progression? How do you as a cancer patient nurture the hope within you or from others?

## Saying Goodbye
For most of us, our inner circle of "loved ones" could include spouses, life partners, children and grandchildren, parents and siblings, and close friends. It is with these individuals that we must face one of the most emotionally difficult tasks saying goodbye. Saying goodbye is not necessarily restricted to the death bed with few moments to spare. For example, while medications can stop being effective, an infection can become critical. Or, if the average life span for a given diagnosis is three to five years, the cancer patient in year one, five years might be all one hears and sounds "pretty good". In year seven for that same patient, the same words can ring like a death knoll.

Another example of reflections by the cancer patient could include what are the words that we use to communicate that we will sooner or later go away and die – meaning being at age 58 years with a five-year life span average might imply that one does not see an infant grandchild graduate from high school, a beloved niece gets married, or a dear friend realizes her dream of becoming an accomplished musician. The challenges of saying goodbye can or cannot evoke powerful reactions and responses for both the cancer patient and the recipient of the message. Emotional preparation for cancer patients and their "inner circles" can be essential for such difficult conversations.

**Living a Meaningful Life**

Living a meaningful life is important for all of us and is especially important for cancer patients. As all cancer patients know, the disease will quickly destroy meaning in one's life as we attempt to cope with an all-encompassing disease. Understanding this process is vitally important for the successful treatment of the disease. We need to come to terms with the fact that the cancer has changed much about who we are; it robs the prior meaning we had about who and what we are, at least to some measure. Bearing this in mind, we have the knowledge and ability to reach within ourselves and recreate who and what we once were. Recognizing that meaningfulness is the cornerstone upon which we rebuild our lives post-diagnosis is the very first step in this process.

**Epilogue - Lessons Learned**

David W. Persky will provide an end summary of all six perspectives. Included in this end summary will be a section on Lessons Learned based upon the author's and contributors' commentaries.

# Meet the Authors

In addition to the senior author Richard E. Farmer, the others include Cindy Bowden, Linda Devine, Diane Linick, Lori Root, Charlie Shockey, Sonja McCaughey, Elizabeth Hapner, and David W. Persky. A brief summary of their professional experiences follows.

Each author will provide an end summary of all five perspectives. Included in this end summary will be a section on Lessons Learned based upon the author's and contributors' commentaries.

In addition to the senior author Richard E. Farmer, a brief summary of their professional experiences follows.

**Richard E. Farmer** is the former President of the Maine College of Health Professions having retired due to his health status with Multiple Myeloma Cancer. Dr. Farmer possess undergraduate degree from Saint Anselm College, a graduate degree from the University of New Haven, and a Doctor of Education degree from Boston University. He is a psychologist, faculty member, and academic administrator. His psychological practice has focused on stress management issues for police, first responders, and government employees. His former presidencies were, as mentioned at the Maine College of Health Professions, at Sanford-Brown College and McIntosh College. He held senior administrative positions at Ohio Dominican University, Saint Leo University, and Providence College. He also held tenured full professorships at the University of New Haven, Sacred Heart University, and Cape Cod Community College. Dr. Farmer is the author of four books, two book chapters, ten refereed journal articles, numerous newspaper articles and professional monographs, and a multitude of research papers presented at professional societies.

**Elizabeth Hapner**
Betsy Hapner is a member of the Florida Bar and the principal of Hapner Law and practices primarily probate and estate planning law. Betsey holds an undergraduate B.A. degree from the University of

Florida College of Arts and Sciences and her J.D. from the University of Florida School of Law. Ms. Hapner is admitted to practice in Florida, before the United States Supreme Court and the Middle District of Florida. She also is an active member of the Hillsborough County Bar Association and the Hillsborough Association of Women Lawyers, where she served as Secretary and as a member of the board for many years. Well known for her commitment to pro bono work, Betsey was honored with the 2022 Jimmy Kynes Pro Bono Service award from the Thirteenth Judicial Circuit, the 2014 Florida Bar President's Pro Bono Service award for the Thirteenth Judicial Circuit and the 2015 Florida's Children First Pro Bono Counsel of the Year award.

Betsey is very active in the Tampa Bay community at large. Among her civic memberships, she is a member of the Economic Club of Tampa, Inc., where she is serving her second term as president; is vice president of the board for the Centre for Women and a member of its League of Extraordinary Women; a former board member of Dress for Success; and the longest serving member of the DUI Counterattack Hillsborough, Inc. She is a member of the Tampa Gator Club and University of Florida Alumni Association, the University of South Florida Women in Leadership and Philanthropy, a former member of the University of Tampa Board of Fellows, the board of the Sulphur Springs Museum and Heritage Center and a member of Mensa. Having lost her son, Kyle to colon cancer in 2020, Betsey is a strong supporter of the Moffitt Cancer Center, one of the leading cancer research centers in the nation.

### Linda Devine

Linda Devine is completing 40 years of service at The University of Tampa, culminating in her current position as Vice President for Operations and Planning, a role that allows her to be a busybody in most areas of the institution while channeling peace. She loves her adopted community and state (although a diehard Browns fan) and has served as president for the Florida Association for Women in Education, Athena Society, Frameworksof Tampa Bay, Inc., and the Rotary Club of Tampa and its Foundation.

Other associations include Leadership Tampa Alumni, Ye Loyal Krewe of Grace O'Malley, and the Junior League of Tampa Community Advisory Board. Linda was selected as 2011 Tampa Bay Businesswoman of the Year in Education and was presented the 2011 Service and Recognition Award by UT's National Alumni Association and NASPA's 2017 Bob E. Leach Award for Outstanding Service to Students. Linda earned a B.S. in education from Ashland College, an M.A. in college student personnel from Bowling Green State University, a Ph.D. in curriculum and instruction from the University of South Florida, and completed Harvard's Institute for Educational Management program. All this is good stuff, but her heart is with her family and friends and time in the garden with her dog, Pizza Marie.

### Diane Linick
Diane Himmel Linick is a retired teacher from Cleveland, Ohio. Diane earned her Bachelor of Science Degree in Education from the Ohio State University (OSU) and her Master of Education, major in Reading K-8 from John Carrol University (JCU). She also earned her certification K-12 LD/BD (Learning Disabled/Behavior Disorder). Diane participated in training about the Deaf Culture and welcomed Deaf/Hard of Hearing (DHH) students and interpreters into her classrooms for many years. As a Reading Specialist she also included ESL students in her specialized small reading groups. Diane has continued her forty years of private tutoring K-12, which is now mainly parent/student ESL and those seeking enrichment.

Diane's teaching experience began at Bellefaire, a residential treatment center for emotionally disturbed children. The school on the grounds was connected to the Cleveland Heights/University Heights (CH/UH) Board of Education. Diane returned to teaching when her two children began school, easing back into teaching as a part time LD/BD tutor at Shaker Heights Middle School. Soon after she became a full-time 3rd grade teacher for The Beachwood City Schools. After receiving her master's degree from JCU she transitioned to the position of Beachwood Elementary School Reading Specialist, where she remained for her last twenty years.

While retired from full-time teaching, Diane has continued with her private tutoring. During the day Diane volunteers at both UH Ahuja Hospital and at InMotion, a wonderful Cleveland nonprofit that provides an array of physical and social/emotional activities and resources for people with Parkinson's Disease and other movement disorders.

### Cindy Bowden

Cindy Bowden was born and raised in the suburbs of Toledo, Ohio and is a first-grade teacher in Granbury, TX. She graduated from Ohio University with a B.S. in communications and was in the graphic design field for 12 years. Cindy was a design artist, assistant editor, desktop publisher, and proposal analyst before shifting career fields. She earned her B.S. in elementary education at the University of North Dakota, graduating summa cum laude. In her public education career, Cindy has taught kindergarten, first, and second grades. She began her teaching career as an alternatively certified kindergarten teacher in Tampa, Florida. Cindy later taught kindergarten in Mabank, Texas and she was nominated for the teacher of the year award. After two years, Cindy transitioned to an early childhood center in Ennis, Texas to teach kindergarten at a new school. At G. W. Carver, she was nominated teacher of the year by her colleagues and received the 2009-10 Kinzie Foundation Award.

After relocating to Corpus Christi, Cindy was hired as a first-grade teacher at Windsor Park Elementary, the International Baccalaureate gifted and talented school in the community. While living in Corpus, she was became a member of Delta Kappa Gamma Society International. In 2018, Cindy accepted a kindergarten teaching position in the Cleburne ISD. During Randall's second cancer battle, she gave up her position mid-year to travel with her deceased husband Randall to MD Anderson in Houston again. While the immunotherapy treatments were working and stopping the progression of the cancer, Cindy took a job as a special education inclusion paraprofessional in the Granbury ISD. Shortly before Randall's death, Cindy was hired by her principal to teach first grade where she currently teaches.

**Charlie Shockey**

Charlie Shockey grew up in Cleveland, Ohio, where he went to high school with co-author Dave Persky, a lifelong friend. Charlie attended Dartmouth College in Hanover, N.H., from 1968-1972, graduating with an A.B., magna cum laude, Phi Beta Kappa, and highest honors in his major. Charlie moved to Washington, D.C. in 1972 and attended Georgetown University Law Center. Soon after graduating in 1975, Charlie met his future wife Irit Arbisser, known to all as Erie. Erie graduated from Georgetown Law two years later. They were married and settled in the Washington, D.C., suburbs of Arlington and Fairfax, Virginia, where they raised their two sons and remained until January 2001, when they moved to Sacramento, California. Charlie's professional career included four positions as an attorney over 37 years, mostly with the Federal Government. He served as an attorney-adviser for the U.S. Department of Energy from 1976-1980, followed by three years in private practice at the Washington Office of a Houston-based law firm, Bracewell & Patterson. In 1983, Charlie returned to the Federal Government as an assistant solicitor in the U.S. Department of the Interior, continuing to work on energy and environmental matters. In 1986, Charlie transferred to the U.S. Department of Justice, where he worked as a trial attorney, senior trial attorney, and assistant section chief in the Department's Environment and Natural Resources Division for the next 27 years, first in Washington, D.C., then in Sacramento. At the Department of Justice, Charlie represented federal agencies and officials in lawsuits concerning environmental laws governing the protection of wildlife and federal lands and resources. Many cases related to the regulation of forests, public lands, national parks, military bases, and water rights. In 2009, Charlie received the Attorney General's Distinguished Service Award and, in 2011, the John Marshall Award, the highest honor given to attorneys at the Department of Justice. He retired in September 2013.

**Sonja (Skyp) McCaughey**

Sonja "Sky" McCaughey is a Hoosier girl from a small town, Berne, Indiana. Her family moved to Florida in 1974 and now considers herself a semi-native Floridian. She grew up in Dunedin and when she graduated from Dunedin High School she moved to Tampa, Florida. Her immediate family consists of two grown children and two grandchildren plus an extended family of four dogs and one squirrel. She currently resides in Inverness, Florida in Citrus County.

She attended Saint Leo University where she received her AA in Liberal Arts and a bachelor's degree in criminal justice. She went through the Tampa police academy, was hired by the Tampa Police Department, and was sworn in as a law enforcement officer on July 29, 1993. In addition to her regular duties, she also served on a multi-agency task force to investigate crimes against children. She later earned her master's degree in criminal justice at Saint Leo and started teaching at Saint Leo University in the Spring of March 2015. She began her doctoral studies at Walden University but left the university to take care of her grandson after her granddaughter was diagnosed with ALL. She retired from law enforcement on October 28, 2016. After teaching for several terms as an adjunct instructor at Saint Leo, she accepted a position as executive director for a ministry that provides specific care for veterans in February 2022.

**David Persky**
David W. Persky is the former tenured full professor of Criminal Justice at Saint Leo University. He holds an undergraduate degree from Southern Methodist University, a master's degree in counseling from Miami University of Ohio, a Ph.D. in Higher Education from Florida State University and Juris Doctorate degree from Stetson University College of Law. Dr. Persky held a variety of administrative and academic positions at the University of South Florida and Saint Leo University. Just prior to his retirement from Saint Leo, he was diagnosed with prostate cancer. He successfully completed radiation therapy and is currently in remission.

David has been highly active in a variety of community service and honor's organizations. He has been a member, president, and district governor for Civitan International. He has served as a volunteer for the Special Olympics, a member of the greater Tampa Chamber of Commerce and a national executive member and

International President for the Kappa Sigma Fraternity. He has been highly active in a number of honor societies including the Alpha Phi Sigma Criminal Justice Honor Society, Who's Who in the South and Southwest, and the Omicron Delta Kappa National Leadership Honor Society. Finally, Dr. Persky received great honors for his work at a number of Florida Universities on the creation and development of a student alcohol abuse program called "My Brother's Keeper".

# Chapter 1:

# Reflections On Caregiving
# To A Cancer Patient

# Change

## By
## Linda W. Devine

It was June 2014. I was sitting in my church, First Reformed Church of Tampa, in my usual way-in-the-back pew, thinking about how good life was. In late April I had relocated my mother from her fifty-plus years in the Ohio countryside to an apartment in the same zip code but in a quintessential charming midwestern town. She was having the time of her life; it was like we had sent her off to college without the homework. My brothers and I were happy that she was experiencing this renaissance well into her 80's.

My thoughts then traveled to my husband Dave. Two of our three children were out of college and in careers they enjoyed, and we were getting ready for a trip to New York City. Our daughter had moved there in 2013, and we enjoyed our short weekend jaunts to the Big Apple, exploring all that it has to offer with our daughter as guide. The promise of interesting food, theatre, walks in great parks, and the never-ending people watching was exciting to me, and, of course, the chance to see our daughter made me exceedingly happy. Life was good.

During our New York trip I noticed that Dave seemed more tired than usual. Our sightseeing occurred in the morning when he was freshest, and then I went on solo explorations in the afternoons, as he wanted to rest in our hotel room. I thought well, he had a busy year teaching, and he needed a break. We often joked about his fourth career – teaching math at Pierce Middle School. It was on a dare from me, a lifer in the educational sector, that he pursues coursework at The University of Tampa. He was an alum, and I serve there as vice president for operations and planning, periodically teaching in the education department. Course after course in education converted him, and he found his new passion in the middle school space. Of course, he was tired!

Teaching seventh and eighth graders was not for the faint-hearted, and summer siestas were warranted. His lethargy seemed nothing more than that, I thought. In late July, he and our longtime friend Jan had decided to try out the Moffitt Cancer Center's new newfangled lung screening equipment. It was advertised in the Tampa Tribune as potential groundbreaking approach to screening for lung cancer. They thought: why not? Both were lifelong smokers, and they were diligent about having regular chest x-rays. In fact, Dave had a chest x-ray in the spring and smoked what would be his last cigarette six months earlier. So off they went to have the Moffitt test, which both he and Jan described as "simple and quick".

One day after Dave's Moffitt screening, he got a call that an oncologist wanted a follow up appointment. We knew that Moffitt had a reputation of responding quickly, and we had an appointment within days of the call. We were concerned, but we countered that with any information derived from the screening would be helpful and that we will "deal with it". During the few days between the call and the appointment we were on a heightened alert. As one who works periodically in emergency situations, I was viscerally responding yet outwardly under control. Dave had enough to ponder, and my partner duties now turned to maintaining "normalcy". We talked to our children, mothers, and brothers, and I re-worked my schedule to give me flexibility. I started to reduce all the questions we had to writing, and I connected individually with all our family members.

This initial triaging responsibility among family and friends was mine, as I made wide berth for Dave to process what might be. He is one of those people that sees the glass half full rather than half empty, and being naturally gregarious, he talked his way through this period, processing out loud. Appointment day - August 6 – arrived. I dressed comfortably and brought a large scarf as hospital settings were often cold for me despite the heat of the Florida summers. I grabbed an old black leather briefcase, placing in it my new notebook filled with a few pages of questions and some of Dave's basic medical information. I drove that morning, a pattern that Dave and I would maintain during all Moffit visits. We started our 30-minute drive in a quiet way, but Dave wanted to review how the visit would be conducted.

We decided I would be the master note taker. I am good at recording as it is part of my profession as an educator to keep track of many things and ask good questions. We talked about the question list and what seemed most important that day. Unlike "normal" Dave, August 6 Dave told me to ask all the questions. I immediately thought that this was not going to happen. I commented that he was a natural talker, and while I would be happy to ask questions, I wanted him to take the lead. He uncharacteristically said that if the news is not great, he would not be able to talk.

We arrived at Moffitt, valet parking which is the Moffit way. This organization always tries to help with the mundane, which I came to fully appreciate months into this journey. We made our path to the thoracic unit that was filled with patients and their people. Dave's name was called, and we moved to Dr. Tawe Taneytown's - "Dr. Tan's" - office. We made small talk for a few minutes, and Dr. Tan stepped into the room. After a kind and brief greeting, he said that the imaging indicated that Dave had stage four lung cancer.

As I heard those words and watched as Dr. Tan brought up the images of Dave's lungs on the computer monitor, I also saw Dave physically change. Rather than his boisterous self, he seemed to have morphed into granite. His face became stone-like and still, his coloring turned to gray, and he was looking somewhere, face slightly cast downward, hands folded in his lap, feet flat on the floor. My observations also included my reaction as I had which I can only describe as an out of body experience. I had heard of such things but was suspicious of their existence, but for the next ten to fifteen minutes I seem to have transposed my consciousness to the upper corner of the room. I watched from behind and above as I asked the questions. I saw myself carefully taking notes, reviewing the notebook list, wrapped in my large scarf. I inquired about the process, the scheduling, the timing, the treatment. While I did not ask him about prognosis, which I knew was less than 19% for a five-year survival rate, I felt comforted by Dr. Tan's hope. I then became fully present in my body as Dr. Tan explained the next steps which would determine the chemotherapy and radiation regimens. Surgery was not an option give the location of the tumors. Dave would qualify for an immunotherapy clinical trial which was showing some promise.

We were left with Dr. Tan's nurse, who took us to see the nutritionist. Dave was somewhat confused by this transition, but it seemed sensible to me as I have always thought of food as medicine. Part of the caregiving would be to have him in the best shape possible for upcoming chemotherapy and radiation which would likely happen contemporaneously. Dave somewhat re-entered the world in this conversation, and he was able to veto cottage cheese and other foods that he disliked as we worked through sample menus.

The 30-minute drive back home turned into two hours as we talked about how we would inform our family. We decided to stop at a Village Inn and ordered breakfast, which neither of us ate. Our conversation focused on our mothers and brothers first, because we knew that those conversations were likely to be easier as we all had life experiences upon which to draw. We devised a strategy to tell our children. I would call their partners first and explain the gravity of the situation. We would then create a conference call with each child and their partner, Dave, and me. In this way everyone would have some support. And we decided that this diagnosis would not be a secret. It is part of our experience, and we can't shield family, friends, colleagues, and others with whom we engage from our new reality.

Our conversations proceeded throughout the afternoon and into the evening, with each person reacting in their own ways of being. We sat in our living room with those that lived locally, and Dave was back into irrepressible the-glass-is-full commentary. He mused, in a matter-of-fact way, that his current situation was the result of a lifetime of smoking, and that he owned that responsibility. He has repeated this often through the years. And while this situation is fraught with deep emotion, Dave only cried when talked about the kids. He had always thought he would see them well into their adulthoods, and now that dream seemed elusive.

Within ten days we had a major readjustment in terms of diagnosis. Dave had a day of testing at Moffitt, including a liver biopsy. I settled into a comfortable Moffitt waiting room, prepared for an afternoon of work on my laptop. A nurse told me that the test had been postponed and that I needed to meet with Dr. Tan and Dave. Upon further examination of the images, it had been determined that his liver was clear of cancer, and that his original stage four diagnosis had been changed to stage three. I recall asking Dr. Tan what all this meant, and I remember the gusto in his voice when he said the "game plan has changed". Dave would still be in a clinical trial with immunotherapy, but it would be coupled with traditional chemotherapy treatments. Radiation would happen contemporaneously. Our odds were now improved, and we left the hospital feeling positive and hopeful.

How life has changed since that quiet June day. Little did I know that I was on a precipice of transformation. I want to say all this change was bad, but I cannot. Dave came through his cancer treatments and on January 6 of the following year was showing no signs of recurrence. He experienced a metastasized brain cancer episode in 2016, but he came through that surgery and radiation. And he was able to work until he decided not to during the Pandemic. We live as normal of a life as we can. We love, we fight, we make up, we go on.

The change that cancer brought was a tangible one, not an esoteric concept. When I heard the diagnosis, a shift in my life occurred immediately. It was palpable and actualized the notion of change in ways heretofore unimaginable and numerous. And this shifting is an odd thing. In my work we talk a lot about reframing conversations, re-positioning, right-siding, and the like, but this shift is like none other. There was a finality to my old life – a good life but a life in which I had not extensive experience with illness nor death. Cancer was the new shifter, the change maker.

# Becoming A Caregiver

## By
## Charlie Shockey

In many respects, I lived a very sheltered and comfortable existence throughout much of the first four decades of my life. I grew up in a modest, middle-class neighborhood on the West Side of Cleveland, Ohio, in the 1950s and 1960s. Maybe not quite Beaver Cleaver, but not far from it. I was fortunate never to have any significant physical or emotional hurdles to overcome. Nor did I have to endure many major family difficulties or tragedies. I was quite unprepared, therefore, to take on the role as a caregiver for a cancer patient, my beloved wife Erie, which I was forced to do starting in 1992 and lasting for the next 25 years. Death and serious illness simply played little role in my young life.

Like most of us, I had limited exposure to, and experience with, the loss of close relatives. My mother's parents both died during the 1950s of heart attack and stroke, respectively, while only in their 60s. My maternal grandmother came to live with my family in 1957, when I was six, and soon thereafter had a stroke that left her partially paralyzed and greatly affected her personality. For the next two years, my parents took my older sister Kate and me to visit grandmother, first in the hospital, then in a nursing home. I have very unpleasant recollections of my first real exposure to her illness and death, based largely on how cranky my grandmother had become following her stroke and then from the sterile and unfriendly atmosphere of the nursing home where she died when I was seven.

I first became a caregiver, in a limited way, a few years later, when my mother had surgery to remove an exceedingly rare tumor from her spinal cord. I was eleven at the time, and my sister and I both knew that her situation was serious, so we were relieved to have her return home and have our lives return to normal. Happily, the tumor was benign, and mom emerged as cheerful and peppy as always. She didn't want or need much care. At the time, I just took everything in stride. Only years later did I learn how potentially serious her prognosis had been.

When I was a teenager and in my early 20s, both my paternal grandparents passed away, from diabetes and prostate cancer, respectively. I knew them reasonably well, as we visited them often in rural western Ohio. I was away at school by the time they died and completely consumed with my own life in college and law school, far removed physically and emotionally from my grandparents in their final years. This was the backdrop for becoming a caregiver for the two most important women in my life.

On the day that Erie and I married in July 1978, my mom told us that she was going in for some medical tests. Three weeks later, when we returned from our honeymoon, we learned the worst possible news. At age 56, she was diagnosed with liver cancer, which had metastasized from her colon. The prognosis was grim, indeed fatal. She was certain to die within a relatively short period of time, and she calmly and bravely accepted that fact. Both Erie and I were devastated. At the outset of our lives together, we knew that we would be deprived of the love and guidance of a truly remarkable woman who touched everyone in her life with acceptance, appreciation, and joy. My mom really was, and remains today, one of the finest human beings I have had the privilege to know.

As mom progressed through chemotherapy in Cleveland, Erie and I would travel back every few months from Washington, D.C., to visit her and share precious time, never knowing if each visit would be the last time. Every departure was tearful and traumatic, as mom bravely and gamely insisted that she would be okay and assured us that so, too, would we. Her attitude made it much easier for the rest of us to cope. She provided a sterling example of how to live with cancer and, when the time came, how to die with dignity.

Her life and death left a lasting legacy that I treasure to this day.

I must admit, however, that I was not responsible as the primary caregiver. That task fell to my older sister Kate, who lived near my mom and who attended every important doctor's visit and hospital test and treatment with her. I regret to say that, due to my living far away and being largely preoccupied with my own life and career, I never fully appreciated all that my sister had to endure during the nineteen months that our mom lived with cancer. Kate, just in her late 20s, provided regular care and companionship and suffered through witnessing mom's decline until her death in February 1980. Not until several decades after my mother's death, did I realize and understand how emotionally difficult the caregiving experience had been for my sister. Because neither Kate nor I ever had to deal with the death of a loved one before our mom died, we were at a loss to know what to do. My mom was not religious and wanted simply to be cremated, with no fuss or ceremony. We honored those wishes, but we were too young and inexperienced to know how to arrange for a memorial service or a fitting and joyful celebration of my mom's life. I deeply regret that failure to this day.

My parents had divorced several years earlier, and my dad remarried and was primarily involved in his own new life. Then, in February 1985, on Erie's birthday, my father died of a sudden, massive heart attack at age 60, shortly after he had retired. Unlike my mother's situation, where we had time to prepare emotionally for her death, my father's death came with no warning. It was beyond surreal to receive a phone call at 6:00 am in a remote part of Alaska in the dead of winter, informing me that my father had died. His wife did arrange for a festive Irish wake in Cleveland one month after he died. It was a fitting way to celebrate his life with his family and friends. And it was exactly the sort of ceremony that I wished we had held for my mom.

All of this was but a prelude to the main event, in terms of my life as a caregiver. Erie and I had settled into our careers and started a family in suburban Washington, D.C., welcoming our son Nathan in 1982 and our son David in 1986. We lived in a comfortable and friendly neighborhood in Fairfax County, Virginia, and the boys thrived with the usual elementary school environment - school, sports, community activities, etc. My days were fully consumed with a combination of family events and work, which often required me to travel around the country as a trial attorney for the U.S. Department of Justice, defending the government in litigation over environmental issues, especially involving protection of wildlife and endangered species. Erie had switched careers from law to social work, which she found far more gratifying. With my busy work and travel schedule, she certainly shouldered more than her share of the child-raising. But we were blessed with a healthy family and a wonderful home life. Until the day that everything changed.

In November 1992, Erie had detected a small lump in her breast at age 39. She had received mammograms regularly, and there was no reason for concern before then, as she had no family history of breast cancer. Her doctor immediately ordered a biopsy of the breast tissue and several lymph nodes. We were frightened and fearful, of course, but we wanted to wait for a more definitive result before sharing the news with our families. The news came as a thunderbolt on the Friday after Thanksgiving. The biopsy revealed that the cancer was malignant, aggressive, and had metastasized to her lymph nodes, which meant that the cancer cells were not confined to the localized breast tissue, but instead had spread elsewhere in her body. We were devastated. Completely. Our idyllic family life was shattered, overnight. Erie assumed the worst. Since the cancer had spread, she was, in her words, "a goner." And I instantly realized that our lives never would be the same and that my role as a husband and father of our two young boys, ages ten and six, would have to change in dramatic ways. Although ill-equipped by both experience and temperament to become a full-time caregiver, I knew that all my attention had to switch to providing all the love and support that I could for Erie and our boys.

We notified our families. As both my parents had died, Erie's family became the focal point of our support network. They were beyond amazing. Her parents and her two brothers, along with their wives, instantly became active and fervent advocates in dealing with the overwhelmingly complex health care system. As her older brother Amir and his wife Lisa were physicians, they were far more knowledgeable than we in knowing whom to call and what questions to ask. We were confident in the care and advice we were receiving from our own doctors, but her family was instrumental in contacting other top-rated cancer clinics around the country, including M.D. Anderson Hospital in Houston, where Erie's parents lived, and the Fred Hutchinson Cancer Center in Seattle, among others.

This was an eye-opening experience for me, to play a vigorous and active role in pressing for details about Erie's condition, exploring all options, and advocating aggressively for the best possible care. The advice we received from the experts around the country was far from uniform, which made the choice of treatment options very difficult. The process of seeking out advice from multiple sources was a new and very transformative one for me. In my own family, we simply trusted our family doctors and accepted their advice without question. Playing a far more active role as Erie's primary caregiver was challenging, but more than worthwhile. The lessons we learned dealing with her medical care and exploring all options would become incredibly valuable two decades later, when Erie's cancer returned.

Erie, thankfully, was greatly buoyed by the support she received from family and friends. We decided early on to be as open as possible about her diagnosis and the treatment options. For us, this transparency in telling everyone about the seriousness of her cancer was comforting. Not everyone approaches cancer and serious illness the same way, of course, but we found that, by letting everyone in on the situation, we were overwhelmed with an outpouring of love and support that we received in return. There were no secrets to keep. Erie's strong, outspoken, hilarious, and unique personality made the darkest days much more bearable for her family, our friends, and certainly for the large complex of medical professionals who suddenly had become an integral part of our lives.

After considering the options, Erie announced that, although the tumor had been found in only one breast, she had decided to undergo a bilateral mastectomy as a preventive measure. In her words, she would "sacrifice both breasts to the breast gods." This was an unusual and somewhat controversial decision in 1992, based on advice from an expert at M.D. Anderson, and Erie's treating physicians at the Fairfax Hospital were somewhat taken aback. But, after extensive consultations, they understood that she knew the risks and was entitled to pursue that course of action. And I, as her husband and caregiver, quickly learned that having lost so much control over her life, she desperately needed to be in control over what she could manage. This was her decision, and she needed me to support her. I did so without reservation.

Following the eight-hour-long and complex surgery to remove both breasts and undergo reconstructive surgery using tissue from her tummy, she emerged exhausted, but relieved. We all remained very concerned for her survival, but also hopeful in knowing that she had so much to live for, especially the future of our young sons. Nate, ten, and very bright and sensitive, readily realized how scary the situation was, as his happy-go-lucky life had been shaken to the core. Dave, not yet six, was far less aware, and we made every effort to keep their lives as normal as possible, given the terrible disruption of seeing their mom in the hospital and throughout the long recovery process.

Following surgery, her oncologist recommended a six-session course of high-dose chemotherapy, to be followed by more than five years on Tamoxifen. The "chemo cocktail," as Erie called it, was incredibly hard to tolerate, and she went through all of the horrible side effects of hair loss, nausea, and diarrhea. Slowly, as the months passed, she began to regain her strength and realize that living with cancer was indeed possible. The hair slowly grew back, and she eventually was able to return to her work as a high school social worker for mentally, physically, and emotionally challenged students, which gave her great satisfaction and a purpose in living beyond that of spending time with family and friends. Life returned to a new normal, and the next years were among the very best and most precious of our lives.

Erie was able to travel again, and we were able to make trips to Israel in 1995 and 2000 to celebrate Nate's and Dave's Bar Mitzvahs at the Western Wall in Jerusalem, surrounded by our loving family. Erie lived with cancer in remission for many years, until 2012, when I would be called on to become her caregiver once more.

# Born to be a Caregiver

## By

## Cindy Bowden

"Randall Bowden, you are an Ironman!" The crowd in Cairns, Australia was cheering, I was screaming, and my husband was grinning from ear to ear after competing for 140.6 miles. Yes, you read that right 140.6 miles. At age 56, Randall swam for just over an hour, biked nearly eight, and then ran a marathon (26.2 miles) in under 5 hours. While he was swimming, biking, and running for over 13 hours, I ate breakfast, wrote post cards, graded papers, ate lunch, took a nap, and then ate dinner. Fast forward 15 months and we're at the doctor's office in Corpus Christi. Did I just hear that right? Did Dr. Mackrizz just say that Randall needed to be hospitalized because "the cancer" is cutting off his kidney and he's one point away from renal failure? We were sitting side by side and I turned to Randall. He had this dazed, questioning look on his face, and in that moment, I took over. I didn't realize it at the time, but I had just become a cancer caregiver for what would be the next five and a half years.

I grew up in Catholic schools, the oldest of four, in a suburb of Toledo, Ohio. My brother Brian and I are two years apart. My younger sisters, Amy and Deidre, were born 9 and 10 years later. I joke that my parents waited to have more children until I was of babysitting-age. I am the responsible one. I set the example for my siblings. And above all, I'm the one looking out for others. Don't get me wrong, this was not dictated by my parents; this thought process was self-imposed. My mom is the heart of our family. She is caring, thoughtful, hard-working, and above all, resilient. Upon high school graduation, I went to her alma mater, Ohio University in Athens, four hours south of where I grew up in Maumee. My parents divorced my freshman year, so looking out for my younger sisters took on a whole new meaning. In 1992, I returned to Toledo, found a job as a graphic artist, and lived close to my mom and sisters during their middle and early high school years. My brother was still attending the University of Toledo.

When the five of us moved to Colorado in June of 1997, I was 27 and ready to take Denver by storm; planning to live with my cousin Tammy. Enter Randall. I met the love of my life just three months later while working as a graphic designer for Denver Public Schools. I believed in love at first sight when I was younger; a real romantic, but had given up hope. Any time he was near I would turn red, a delightful trait we fair-skinned people have, and my heart would race. He truly took my breath away. Tammy jokes that the first time she saw us together she thought to herself, "Well, there goes my roommate..." She was right. Randall was intelligent. He was so handsome and funny. And he was a genuinely good, self-made man. He took on responsibility as a teenager, helping his single Mom by working to pay utility bills for their family of four in southern California. He married at 18 and helped raise two beautiful, intelligent, and strong women; daughters Nikki and Sarah, while working full time and going to college full time to earn his degrees. Randall was everything I love and admire in a person.

We were married in Estes Park, Colorado, on the front lawn of the Stanley Hotel. Randall earned his doctorate and started applying for jobs in higher education. His last words before flying to San Antonio to interview at University of the Incarnate Word: "We're not moving to Texas...this is just interview practice." His words on the phone one day later: "They offered me the job, and they want an answer before I leave tomorrow." Thus, began our adventure together. They don't tell you that when you marry a professor, it's like being in the military. Randall needed to be challenged, and move up and on throughout his career. We've lived in Colorado, Florida, North Dakota, and Texas. Most recently we moved to Granbury, where Randall took a position at Tarleton State University. This was our fourth move within Texas, having lived in Corpus Christi, at Cedar Creek Lake (east of Dallas), and in San Antonio. Randall, our black lab Sami, and I were a family! We moved around the country together and for the first time in my adult life, someone else was loving and taking care of me, just as much as I was loving and caring for him.

Now, back to September 2016. I realized immediately that my number one role as cancer caregiver was to help him fight for his life. My first step was contacting MD Anderson Cancer Center in Houston every day for (what ended up being) three weeks until they consented to see Randall. I was relentless; calling up to 5-6 times a day, waiting on hold to talk to or be transferred to employees in several departments. Once you become a patient at MDA, you're in capable hands; the medical professionals there are the leaders in their field, creating individualized cancer treatment plans for every patient. However, getting an initial appointment at MDA is one of the toughest jobs I'd ever faced. Randall's first biopsy results were inconclusive and the second biopsy was misdiagnosed. His biopsy and blood work from Dr. Mackrizz in Corpus Christi bounced from department to department at MDA in Houston until the paperwork landed on Dr. Arlene Siefker-Radtke's desk. Those three weeks were agony; waiting and wondering what would happen next. Would Randall start feeling sick? Would he die because he wasn't getting treatment? Would the doctors be able to treat the cancer? Had it spread so much that he wouldn't be able to survive it? One thing was for sure—he did have stage 4 cancer. Randall went from competing 140.6 miles in Australia in June of 2015 to having stage 4 cancer in September 2016; passing stages 1-3. He had no symptoms until September 11, 2016, when he couldn't stop throwing up at a Houston 70.3 triathlon. To say that we were shocked Randall had cancer, albeit stage 4 cancer, was an understatement. He was one of the healthiest people we knew. He had 4.5% body fat. He biked 60 miles and ran half-marathons to train for that 140.6-mile competition, for Pete's sake!

I was on sabbatical from teaching and now focused on Randall beating cancer. We drove to Houston for doctor's appointments, PET scans, CT scans, blood work, and chemotherapy treatment. Because it was stage 4 and spread throughout the trunk of his body, his oncologist, Dr. Siefker-Radtke, created a brutal treatment plan. We drove to Houston on Monday morning for Randall to have blood work. He was admitted to the MDA hospital Monday afternoon, where he was given 4 hours of chemotherapy and then 16 hours of fluids to flush the poison through his system. This went on for 5 days. We checked out of the hospital on Saturday. Randall had two weeks "off" in between treatments where he continued to work for Texas A&M Corpus Christi (TAMUCC). He was hospitalized at MDA a total of four times with this week-long chemotherapy treatment. Dr. Radke said she would have to "take him down to nothing" in order to beat the cancer. The only reason he was able to have this harsh, extreme treatment is because he was already in such good shape physically. I stayed with Randall in his room during those four separate treatment weeks. He was poked and prodded all day and all night. The nurses wore hazmat suits when they brought and administered one of the bags of chemotherapy. Randall was in his gown and I sat and watched in my pajamas. By April of 2017 Randall was cancer free. Thank you to the angels in scrubs at MD Anderson in Houston!

No one knows the emotional roller coaster that is cancer unless they've lived it. Protocol for cancer survivors is having PET scans for up to five years after treatment. Randall and I drove back to Houston every three months, praying and holding our breath, for a scan to reveal that he was still cancer-free. On his 12-month scan, Dr. Siefker-Radtke saw a small spot in his pelvic bone. When we returned three months later, the spot was larger so she sent Randall to have it biopsied. He had a second cancer, again, stage four. Yes, you read that right. In August of 2018, he developed stage 4 cancer in just 3 months. I remember sitting there in her office, when she told us about finding cancer, again, and feeling dazed. Randall took one look at my face and said, "what's next?" My disbelief turned to an anger so intense, I think we were both surprised by it! This was not supposed to happen again. Randall went through treatment and the cancer was gone. He wasn't supposed to go through that brutal chemotherapy treatment and suffer through those horrific side effects to be diagnosed with a second cancer. He beat the cancer. It's gone. I said very little. Randall's next question was, "Can I compete in an Ironman in Kentucky in October?" Ironically, he'd been training over the last 9 months to enter a second, "I kicked cancer!" 140.6-mile competition. The doctors told him to "listen to his body" while training because, again, he had no symptoms.

To say that our reactions to this cancer news was opposite of our reactions in 2016 was an understatement! Randall seemed unphased and took charge; I was angry and in denial for some time to come. "Stage 4 metastatic melanoma has no cure and a 20% remission rate." These are the words I seemed to hear time and again in my head over the next two and a half years. My role as cancer caregiver would last the rest of Randall's life.

# On Being A Cancer Caregiver

## By

## Diane Linick

Family dynamics often change during a cancer journey. As the caregiver I needed and wanted to respond calmly to my loved ones to meet their constantly changing emotions and physical needs. I promised my husband David that I would "follow his lead" to navigate this new and unsettling phase of our life. I wish to share a little background of our history to explain how unexpectedly and involuntarily exchanging our roles made David's journey rough beyond his physical pain. He loved to give to others. Over the years he often told me that he loved being a father and a husband. He went out of his way to do for us. He truly enjoyed giving of himself as our family leader and he was our role model.

We were the exception of the many college freshmen couples we knew, as we were able to study together and date at the same time! We brought the best out in each other. His parents credited me with his becoming the high achiever they always knew he could be and I appreciated and needed his organization and calming demeanor for the rigors of studying and mainly time management. Preceding our senior year of college, we married. Following graduation David went on to law school. Making important long-term goals about our education, our career plans, and family life, established our ability to respect each other's opinions and needs while still in college. We were mutually private about family issues, health, and finances with others. Together we discussed family decisions large and small. Little did we know that a cancer diagnosis would present a slight crack in our view of how to deal with each other's concerns.

This privacy issue became quite difficult for me from the beginning. In the car ride home from the initial visit with the oncologist, I repeated that I would "follow his lead" with respect for all of his needs and wishes throughout his journey. My first question was, "How do we tell our children?" He was firm in his mind that our children should know exactly what the doctors told us that day and throughout treatment. I assumed we would tell everyone the basics of the diagnosis and what immediate tests were scheduled. I especially felt Amy and Brian needed a little time to adjust to their dad's diagnosis. David responded with a stoic "no". I was somewhat shocked at this response. On the other hand, David did not want me to relay his medical reports to other than closest family and friends. He left no room for discussion, unusual for us. (I would learn in the following months why such a strong reaction.) He was adamant that they were not to be given any false hope. He did not want his identity to become " cancer patient" to his friends and business contacts. I tried one small compromise and offered that we could tell them the diagnosis and test results needed first and then tell the prognosis as treatments and trials took place.

I've always been the one overly concerned about safety and emotional/physical well-being of all members of our family. He thrived on being the family home and financial manager, loving father, and husband. David especially respected my knowledge of childhood development in both home and school etc. He was the family confidant due to his respected problem solving and legal skills. Our extended family regarded him to be fair and gracious with his ability to listen and always use sound judgment. In short, we had always "depended" on him. It was extremely difficult, but he soon realized that he had to "depend" on me as his primary caregiver. David's "work" routines stayed in place through remote communications. It was most disappointing for him to slowly relinquish his responsibilities at home. I was honored, yet constantly worried that I was not meeting all of his needs, while at the same time respecting his independence, even as it waned.

Driving my husband to and from places when he was weary from all things cancer was a perfect example of this. (I have never been comfortable when driving outside of familiar areas or on the freeways). These trips were unsettling for both of us. Just having tests, appointments with new specialists in addition to his lead doctor and worrying about possible new treatment side effects produced anxiety before getting in the car. We were content with our usual roles as David the driver and me the passenger. I felt responsible for his unease and irritability before even entering a medical center. The last thing I wanted to do was make a difficult day worse, especially when my goal was to make David as comfortable as possible.

I have been involved in caregiving as a wife, mother, daughter, and sister. I learned that each family member and student had different needs of my time during their care. I could even sense when certain strengths of mine were helpful, such as being a quiet companion at home or in the hospital or listening to and validating their emotions and fears. I became a strong advocate at appointments and especially in the hospital for treatment or an inpatient stay. I have used this new strength to care for others as well as myself. My note taking skills were depended on during my husband's, sister's, and parent's medical appointments, tests, treatments, plus ER and inpatient stays. What they didn't know was that doing something during tough appointments was more helpful to me. It kept me focused and became a journal for us both. Most days David would want me to read these notes aloud. This request made me feel I was doing exactly what he wanted me to do. From these notes David was better able to stay involved and form questions about his test results and care plan. These routines were also helpful to my other family members. It seemed like they felt somewhat in control of their care whenever I reviewed the doctors' comments. We worked as a team, and we learned together.

I find it hard even now to mention any of my challenges and thoughts about being a caregiver. How could I even think to myself for a second how exhausting working full time and trying to be there for family members including my spouse, children, siblings, parents and even students simultaneously? It was heartbreaking to hear apologies from my loved ones for.

having cancer invade our lives and being so needy of my time I didn't share their view. I loved being with them and grateful to be "their person" in all ways needed. However, I felt guilty being the healthy one. I did not dwell on that but used it as personal motivation to do whatever it took to make each of them my top priority.

I am pleased to share that I enjoyed the special individual times with each of my loved ones. David's pride in taking care of his family gave him great satisfaction. At the same time I think we both knew that some changes in family responsibilities would affect our emotional state, each in a different way during phases of treatments. We each had days when we felt as if we had failed one another. He became depressed and I felt stressed on so many levels. After we got into a routine these feelings of resentment toward cancer and its effects faded slightly.

For David, resting with him while he was napping or sitting quietly each evening in his office or in a hospital room was comforting for him as well as me. As one of my sister's caregivers I realized that I could be most helpful through our evening phone calls. Ellen loved spending her days with her family and wonderful friends. With me she needed to share her day's frustrations and fears before she went to bed. Selfishly I needed private time with Ellen. Quietly sitting with David and having sister time with Ellen each evening came to be some of my most beautiful memories. I was honored and appreciative that both my husband, sister and parents felt extremely comfortable with me as one of their special caregivers. I even came to understand that I was their trusted sounding board. That role often was as a punching bag, a release for their frustrations during the journey. I assured them I understood and even encouraged them to vent! Patients need a chosen person, their caregiver, to be there for them during the hardest of times to share with you their fears, hopes, anger, discomfort, and frustration with Cancer. I hoped every day that I provided some form of comfort.

# I Am Grammie, A Cancer Caregiver

## By

## Sonja McCaughey

*"Mom, I need your help."*

I was in the office working on yearly evaluations for my squad mates in the Tampa Police Department (TPD). The call came in the afternoon in August of 2016 to my cell phone. When I saw that my son was calling me and knowing that he was in Germany, I quickly went to an area within the Tampa Police District Two office where the reception would not be interrupted during the phone call. When I answered the call, I immediately heard in my son's voice that something was wrong.

My son was serving in the U.S. Army and was on assignment in Germany but was deployed to Poland. My daughter-in-law, grandchildren, and grand puppy were in Germany at the time I received his call. I live in the United States.

Very quickly and with disbelief and sadness in his voice he told me that his daughter was just diagnosed with leukemia, and they would be leaving Germany, flying directly to the Walter Reed Medical Center within 48 hours. My son asked me if I could please meet them at the airport and get them to the hospital. The doctors would be waiting for her arrival to start treatment immediately. He also stressed that his wife needed my help too.

As I was talking to my son, Lieutenant Kurt Rojka of TPD entered the area and could hear the difficult, stressed conversation. When I hung up the phone Lt. Rojka asked me if everything was okay. I told him no and that I needed to leave to help my son. Lt. Rojka heard most of the conversation and I filled in what he would need to know. Police officers don't cry at times like this. We become stoic because we are trained to help those in crisis. Within minutes my round-trip flight was being paid for by my Lieutenant. Lt. Rojka's actions humble me to this day as this was the first time that I could remember somebody doing something for me in a crisis moment, without asking anything of me in return. I quickly put in notice with TPD that I needed to take vacation time, hired a pet sitter to take care of my four dogs, and prepared myself to be gone for a week before I started to absorb the shocking reality that my 9-year-old granddaughter, Nikita, was now a cancer patient. I knew my immediate role and that was to meet them at the airport. I called my son back and assured him that plans were in motion, and I would pick them up at the airport.

My mind was racing on the flight to Washington about my granddaughter and how was I going to be a cancer caregiver for her and my son's family. I have never been called up for this kind of role and I was not sure how I was supposed to support my family. I needed to remind myself of my position of being a grandmother and wanted answers to so many questions as my family was in a crisis mode.

I learned that my daughter-in-law had taken Nikita and her younger brother to a water theme park in Germany. They were there for about five hours, jumping on trampolines and enjoying the water park. The next morning my granddaughter woke up and complained of a sore ankle. My daughter-in-law is a good mom and quickly responded with "What do you expect? You were jumping on a trampoline for five hours your ankle probably is sore." My granddaughter is incredibly smart. She was taking piano lessons, she was on a competitive gymnastics team, and a ferocious tomboy; joint injuries are common in these types of activities. She was a daredevil and did not have any fear of trying anything. But after a week of her complaining about her ankle my daughter-in-law decided to take her to a pediatrician to find out why her ankle was sore. Her ankle was x-rayed, and Nikita did not have any breaks or stress fractures. The pediatrician could not press on anything that would indicate soreness or pain. The pediatrician then decided to do some blood work just as a precautionary measure. A couple of days later the blood work came back and Nikita's white blood count was extremely high. The official diagnosis: Acute Lymphocytic Leukemia - ALL.

Cancer treatment is evasive to anybody, especially for a young child whose neurological system and brain are not fully developed. The military made it very clear that it would not allow another country to treat this cancer. It was decided that Nikita would be flown immediately to the Walter Reed Medical Center and treatment would begin as soon as she arrived.

Day 1. My daughter-in-law's mother was staying with the family in Germany when Nikita's cancer diagnosis was made; she lived in South America. The decision was made to leave my four-year-old grandson and the dog in Germany with the other grandmother while my daughter-in-law and granddaughter flew back to the United States while my son continued his deployment in Poland. The flight was 15 hours long and both Nikita and her mother arrived exhausted from the flight; exhausted from having to uproot their home; exhausted with the unknown of the journey that they were about to begin. I met them at Ronald Reagan International Airport (Reagan) and we drove to the Walter Reed Medical Center where the medical team was waiting for us. We arrived around 11:30 P.M. I remember the kindness of the nurses who were dealing with three very exhausted ladies who were hungry, tired, overwhelmed with the information about cancer, and scared.

The first procedure was to draw blood and my granddaughter had lost all of her patience a long time ago. I had never heard Nikita scream like that before in my life. She did not understand that she had cancer. She did not understand the nurses needed to draw her blood so that they could start her treatment to battle cancer. She did not understand why her mom and her Grammie were not helping her. But those experienced nurses understood, and they gave her time to calm down and fluids to keep her hydrated. The nurses decided to numb her skin before any more needles were going to be used on her. They spoke directly to Nikita, not around her, not over her, but to her face so that she understood what they were going to do and when they were going to do it. My granddaughter absorbed those words with intense eyes on them. I prayed hard to God that the numbing medication worked so they would not have to stick her again.

Her mother and I stepped out of the room to give the nurses the much-needed control to deal with Nikita. It is hard to leave when you hear fear screaming from a little girl. My prayers were answered. My daughter-in-law was trying extremely hard to be strong; however, she was exhausted, and rightfully so. Exhausted from the 15-hour flight and exhausted that she was away from her four-year-old son, away from her husband, and having to leave them in two other countries to take care of a sick child. The nurses had a lot of work ahead of them in remaining calm with this exhausted chaos that was going on.

Where do I fit in?

Day 2. Fortunately, my granddaughter was able to get some much-needed sleep; however, her mom and I were physically exhausted but mentally alert as we watched and observed all the nurses and doctors that came into the room. So many doctors and so many nurses walked into that room, and I will always remember that they brought staff that would educate my granddaughter on what was going on with her body and what kind of treatment she was going to get. Even a dietician came in to brief us on the importance of eating healthy and what foods would make it harder for her body to go into remission. The amount of knowledge and intelligence that came into our room was overwhelming. It was time for a crash course on cancer. It was time to learn what kind of cancer Nikita had and how this cancer was going to be treated. Lab results were written on a board, and they were regularly updated so that everyone could see the fluctuation of the lab results of when medicine was working.

I am still wondering, where do I fit in?

Day 3. The hospital brought in support staff for the family. What was impressive is they brought in material that my granddaughter could understand. They had books with detailed pictures of what all components of her blood looked like. They brought in medical equipment and explained what the equipment was and how it was going to be used on her. They explained when it would hurt and when it would not hurt. They allowed her to ask as many questions as she needed to, and they answered her in terms she understood. They allowed her to have as much control over a situation that she had no control over as possible. This was empowering for Nikita because once she understood her internal chaos settled down. If she was calm, we all were calmer. I was so impressed by how the staff made sure Nikita understood what she had and how it had to be treated. They were strong advocates for her and would not allow us to interfere with any explanation – this was not their first cancer patient.

I still have no idea what I am supposed to be doing?

Day 4. My son arrived from Germany and finally made it to the hospital. He was exhausted and we bombarded him with medical information within 20 minutes of his walking into the room. Nikita was happy to see her daddy. The good news was that Nikita's white blood count was coming down and the treatment that she was receiving was working. My son confirmed her questions and that she was going to be okay. That is all she needed to hear. It was at this point that we all took a deep breath and began to discuss our future. Although this was a family matter, and I know my place as Grammie; the Army was to make important decisions about my family's future as well as Nikita's parents.

I am confused, do I need to be here?

Day 5. My grandson and grand puppy were still in Germany. The decision was made to have my grandson stay with his aunt in Belgium because his other grandmother was going back home to South America. The grand puppy would be cared for by a family in Germany. I felt so helpless because my son was going to go back to Germany in a couple of weeks to pack up the entire home to be shipped back to the United States. He would need help coordinating the logistics of the move to fly back to the United States with his son in Belgium and the family dog in Germany, however, he is Army strong. I felt helpless because I didn't know whom I could help the most at this moment. My son made the decision for me to stay with his daughter at Walter Reed Medical Center until it was time for me to go back home.

My sweet Nikita was diagnosed with ALL at the age of 9. At this early stage of the diagnosis of her illness, since the leukemia was discovered fast, we were told that she would have a high success rate for cancer to go into remission. However, there was a 17 to 25 percent chance the cancer would return when she was in her early twenties, and it would be aggressive. She would be with an oncologist for a very long time. This type of cancer hides really well in the body. Even though lab results were looking positive we were told that one tiny cell may be hiding in her body and her treatment would be aggressive. The doctors were very familiar with this cancer, and they knew how the treatment plan was going to occur.

Day 6: The army of doctors came into Nikita's room and informed us that she would need an implanted port. It was the best answer for reducing the invasion of containments into her body by the many injections she would need as well as giving her the medications needed without additional needles. The nurses would use this port to draw blood as well as give her medication. The process was explained: the port was small and would be implanted under her skin but that we could see the port. There would be a line that would go into one of her veins and giving medication and drawing blood would not be painful for Nikita. My granddaughter was going to surgery to have a port put into her body. She was so little. The doctors were worried because she was petite and wondered whether she had enough skin to cover the port and whether it would stay in place. Placing the port would be important for several reasons. We asked many questions about just the port. How big is the port? Where will it be put in? How long will she have the port? What happens if the port malfunctions? Will the scar eventually fade so it would not be noticeable as she grew older? I remember hearing the port can stay up to ten years if needed. TEN YEARS!? One nurse made the comment that the port will leave a scar but when Nikita puts on her wedding gown it will be faded. At that moment, those words made me smile and I think at that moment I finally took a deep breath.

The surgery was successful. However, nausea struck hard. The nurses held Nikita's long hair back as she threw up and reassured her; she would be okay. I saw her nod her little head.  She had a hard time coming out of the anesthesia until one of the nurses put a popsicle to her lips.

My granddaughter is a daddy's girl. She needed her father to be with her. My son was a career military man, and he was doing the best he could to be with her. I am Grammie. I know my place. I could not take control of my son's family and I could not take control of this cancer. But as a caregiver for my granddaughter, I could be there for whatever they needed, but it was time for me to go back home.

# Initial Diagnosis

## By

## Elizabeth Hapner

Nothing can ever prepare you for the words "Mom, I have cancer" or "Your son has Stage 4 colon cancer." In that instant, life changed forever. Words are inadequate to describe just how devastating that news was. My son, and only child, Kyle was thirty years old when we received the fateful diagnosis on June 18, 2018. When I arrived at St. Joseph's Hospital in Tampa, across the street from where I had given birth to Kyle, I learned that he had more than one million cancer cells. His condition was deemed terminal from diagnosis, but we did not give up hope, particularly with the advances in treatment that kept being developed. As horrific as the news was, my focus immediately became taking the best possible care of my child and having the greatest possible quality of life together for the time he had remaining.

By way of background, my son had been suffering from abdominal pains for more than a year. Thirteen months earlier, Kyle called to tell me that he was in the Emergency Room of a local hospital and had been told that he had appendicitis. His appendix was removed that day and he was hospitalized for three days. Ironically, I had to rush from the memorial service of a good friend who had just died of colon cancer to the hospital to pick him up upon his release. Despite the appendectomy, he continued to experience the same pain over the coming months.

Kyle returned to the emergency room and to the doctors to whom he was referred over the course of the next year. He was told he had either ulcerative colitis or diverticulitis but was never placed on medication for it or referred for a colonoscopy. I told him a number of times that he needed to see someone else. Finally, one

Monday morning, he was in such pain at work that he went to a different emergency room, resulting in the fateful diagnosis. It was just eleven days since he had been in the emergency room of the initial hospital when he was finally properly diagnosed. The sole outcome of the last emergency room visit to the first hospital was that they finally ordered a colonoscopy, to take place in mid-August. Undiagnosed and untreated, we were told Kyle would not have survived long enough to ever have that scheduled colonoscopy.

Kyle's situation should never have occurred. But for malpractice, his cancer would have been diagnosed early enough for successful treatment. The removal of his appendix caused his colon to shift, and the tumor then fused his upper and lower colon, making it inoperable. By the time of his diagnosis, it had spread to his liver. My belief is that they failed to consider cancer as a possibility because of his young age and because they were predisposed to believe that any young person presenting with pain was simply seeking prescription pain medications.

Coming to terms with Kyle's diagnosis was an arduous task. Needless to say, the most difficult part was the eventual acceptance that his situation was fatal. Second was accepting the fact that it never should have been a death sentence for him and that we had no recourse against the health care professionals who had repeatedly committed malpractice in their care of him. Kyle and I were determined that the remainder of his life would be as meaningful as possible and that we would spend as much quality time together as was possible.

I was shocked to learn of the significant increase in cancer cases among young adults. The percentage of people under recommended screening age with colorectal cancer has increased fifty-one percent since 1994. Colorectal cancer is the number one cancer in young men while breast cancer is first for young women. Half of those young adults with colorectal cancer were obese. Kyle was always a healthy person, playing ice hockey, basketball and other sports and was not overweight. Chemicals and pesticides have been identified as major factors in the spread of cancer in young adults.

Caregiving for an adult child with cancer obviously differs from that of a younger child with cancer but many of the tenets are the same. Because my son was an adult, living independently, I was unaware of just how extreme the pain was that he was suffering, prior to his diagnosis. He also was the one in charge of all decisions concerning his treatment, a difficult position for any parent to accept when the consequences of any decision could be so significant. My job was to be there to support him, offer advice and care for him in his last weeks. At times, this was far easier said than done. Someone with a younger child with cancer faces a somewhat different set of challenges in caregiving, as does someone whose child is not terminal. Everyone's journey is different.

Armed with Kyle's diagnosis, we began the journey through treatment. The first week was spent in the hospital where he was diagnosed, going through further testing and putting in a port. Kyle was initially resistant to the idea of a port but when he learned how frequently he would be subjected to needles in his veins, he quickly changed his mind. (Kyle had always had a fear of needles.) This was just the first in a long series of decisions that I had to approach in an indirect fashion to convince him of the best decision.

The first week brought lots of tears, from both of us and from other family and friends. I had to be careful to balance emotions with the necessary strength to support his needs. Kyle was never one for much outward emotion, but this was the most traumatic news of his life, so he did give in to the overwhelming rush of sorrow and fear. More traumatic even than the initial diagnosis was the subsequent news that his condition was deemed inoperable and that he had a life expectancy of just a year. Kyle had watched his close friend, Matt, suffer through a lengthy battle with cancer to which he had succumbed four years before Kyle's diagnosis.

Every step of the journey was a learning experience. We had never dealt with cancer in our family before. Once we got through the trauma of the initial diagnosis, Kyle's first concern, aside from dying, was that he did not want to lose his hair. The type of chemotherapy he underwent did not involve hair loss.

As an attorney, I am accustomed to the fact that my profession tends to speak a different language than the general public. Now it was my turn to learn a new language. Many acronyms and unfamiliar medical terms are used in oncology. In order to understand blood tests results, we had to learn what each listing was and what the numbers indicated.

One of the first learning experiences was when it came time for Kyle to come home from the hospital. Before he could be released, I had to have his pain medication prescriptions filled. The hospital pharmacy did not carry such narcotics for use outside the hospital. I went to a local pharmacy to fill the prescriptions, only to learn that they would not fill them. It took trips to five different pharmacies before the prescriptions were filled. Meanwhile, my child was anxiously awaiting his release to come home to my residence.

The day after Kyle's release from the hospital we had an outpatient appointment with the group that had been treating him in the hospital. It was then that we were told definitively that his life expectancy was no more than a year. The previous evening, I had contacted our local national cancer institution to arrange for him to be seen there. It would take over a week before an appointment would be set for him to be seen there as I was required to have records sent for review before they would assign doctors to see him. The process of gathering records, including CDs of his scans, was time-consuming both in terms of my time and the amount of time it took for them to prepare the records.

Approximately ten days later, we had our initial appointment at the local national cancer institution, Moffitt Cancer Center. We were fortunate to be given a representative to guide us through the initial process. The facility was so large, and so unfamiliar, that it was overwhelming. Her guidance was priceless. Despite that, it was too much to process, both in terms of the amount of information and finding our way around the physical plant. The initial appointment was with the oncologist who would be assigned to treat Kyle. The ultimate decision as to where he would be treated was Kyle's, but I was relieved when he decided to treat at Moffitt. We were very comfortable with the oncologist there. We went on to an appointment with the surgeon who was assigned to evaluate whether surgery would be an option. That surgeon met with a complex case treatment team to make that decision. In retrospect, I wish I had insisted on more information early on.

Although the complex treatment team considered the possibility of surgery on several occasions, it was rejected each time. I was not aware, until a year later, that Kyle had responded to chemotherapy as well as he did the first few months. The assigned surgeon did not convey this information to us and we were still navigating the learning process as far as both terminology and the website for the cancer center. Had I known just how low his levels had dropped by the time the treatment team evaluated the possibility of surgery for the second time, I would have taken Kyle to M.D. Anderson at the time for a second opinion.

# Chapter 2:

# Obtaining Support

# The Round Table

## By
## Linda W. Devine

I remember sitting at Village Inn in Tampa, Florida. It is a humble gathering place for people from all walks of life, an affordable restaurant where we could grab eggs and toast and pancakes when the kids were small. "VI" was a common meeting place for pedestrian coffee and a slice of pie.

It was early April of 2015, and Dave my husband had just run through the gauntlet of chemotherapy and radiation during the previous fall. He had a great medical visit in January, with a "keep doing what you are doing" prescription from his thoracic physician at Moffitt Cancer Center. This period was tempered by Mom's poor health; she had been convalescing in a beautiful facility on the south shores of Lake Erie, and I flew up as often as reasonable, keeping my work and Dave's schedules synced. It was time to bring her to Florida, something we had always planned, even in her healthy days.

Dave and I had agreed early in our marriage that we would do this for our parents, regardless of the circumstances. My Dad had passed in 1993, and she reiterated that she wanted to live with me "when the time came". And the time had come. It was at that round table at Village Inn that I began my caregiver support journey in earnest. During Dave's treatment in the previous year, I was able to handle most of the stressors as he tolerated chemotherapy and radiation treatments fairly well. Although the appointments seemed never-ending, providing nutritious meals, managing medications, and making sure he had good social connections were things that I could do with some facility. He was ambulatory, could drive, and chatted nonstop with friends and family. He was good at letting me know what was troubling him, and our circles of friends and family made the tasks manageable.

But this round table encounter - and the intervention that it came to be now that I see it from a distance – was different. Mom was 86, on dialysis, and had contracted the chloridoids difficile infection ("C. diff) while at the rehab facility. This gathering was different. I was already a cancer caregiver, and now this role had been extended to caring for Mom, a person who had done much during her life to ensure that my brothers and I moved into adulthood with a toolkit of values and skills that would serve us well. I felled compelled to hold up my obligation to her, and to do it well, giving her a quality of life that she deserved.

The gathering was one I had engineered but in hindsight, the women present were waiting for my call. The group consisted of my friends at First Reformed Church of Tampa, where I had attended services since the late 1980's. Present were nurses: Peg, who was known at St. Joseph's Hospital as the person who ran the facility at night. Meredith was a nurse, and in her retirement, she is the nexus of church's prayer chain, a collection of folks who learn the needs of others and commit their needs to prayer and meditation. Viva was there, too: she and I raised our kids together at First Reformed, and her specialty area was geriatric nursing, although she had since switched up and managed quality assurance programs for a large company. Sandy, the Church administrator sat with me, too. Her practicality and midwestern sensibility always fueled my soul. And my dear mother-in-law, Elaine, was at the table, as always. Saint Elaine, I should add, as she raised five fine sons and led a quiet life of service that was legendary in our community.

These women sat with me as I described my mother's medical maladies as best as I could in lay person terms. I shared how the personnel at the beautiful Ohio facility seemed more interested in moving her out than helping me find permanent solutions. That maybe I hoped for too much, and asked the wrong questions. It was at that round table that I tried to look brave and confident because - - well, I manage things wonderfully at work, and why should this be any different? I solve complex problems every day. I know how to marshal resources to a common good. My friends patiently listened to me, and then the gentle questions began. They were not commentaries about how I should do things but rather kind probing about how I could get from point A to point B. I did not know how to schedule skilled assistance for Mom. I was overwhelmed with the lists of agencies that I had been handed by medical personnel. My good friends pointed out that solutions existed in our congregation. A couple we knew ran a senior assistance program targeting just the kind of help that Mom needed. I had seen a presentation they had conducted some months prior and simply did not connect the dots, likely because I was on information overload.

There were other round tables of support that happened. I understand now that my five longtime girlfriends were worried about how I could handle a full-time job, a husband who had had early success with cancer treatment, and now a mother who needed me. They knew my time would not be my own.  Even with a caregiver covering 40 hours a week, there were still another 128 hours that I needed to manage. The round tables we experienced were ad hoc: a meal on a Friday evening while Dave stayed with Mom, a boat trip across the bay on a Saturday when I could get coverage. In many respects they were normalizing my life, providing respite through laughing and chatting about our families and work.

In those hours I was free, engrossed in whatever gabfest they launched. My round table activities extended to my closest work colleagues, both local and remote. Some of those times were shared over Mexican or Thai lunches as they helped me figure out work plans. Each had their own hectic work and family life, yet they found ways to support my responsibilities. Some of those conversations extended to evening Zoom calls that were scheduled every three to four weeks, always around my schedule as I had the least time options to offer. Again, my colleagues were always good about checking in with me, something that I naturally do with others. Yet I was somewhat uncomfortable when asked how I was doing.

I was very good at providing quick, affirmative responses and then sailing on to how others were doing. This group in particular would stop me cold at the doorway of conversation and plumb the depths of how I was really faring. They did not accept the "fair to middling'" response I might give, and they would comment on how I seemed tired, distracted, or whatever the day had brought. This would be a precursor, now that I can look backward, to what would be important in the years to come.

These support groups coalesced in a mighty way in the spring of 2016 when Dave's cancer had metastasized to his brain. Although this was an "easy" surgery according to the physicians, it was a setback that seemed to come from nowhere. Our circle of support rallied. Rich, one of Dave's golfing and teacher friends, made sure he had company until the wee hours of the morning so I could be home to tend to Mom. Dave's brothers rallied around him, taking turns to make sure he stayed focused on his recovery. Our kids popped in and out, bringing comic relief. And the First Reformed Prayer chain and many text groups were in full force.

Looked back on the networks of support I had as a caregiver, I am now struck by how my strengths could quickly turn to liabilities if not managed. According to Gallup's Strengths Finder, a widely used instrument that assesses 34 strengths, my top five signature strengths are Achiever, Learner, Input, Relator, and Responsibility. As one who embodies Achiever and Responsibility, my nature is such that I am task driven and have the stamina to work hard. This, when paired with my need to fulfill my obligations in a quality way, is a road to burnout. I suspect Team Linda saw that in me and hence circled their wagons around me when they could. I am driven to care, and I see that as an obligation to my family. And my Learner/Input/ Relator is a triad of strengths that makes me naturally seek help.

My inquisitiveness and natural bent to learn from others likely opened doors for me. I sought knowledge from those who could provide it, solace from my mindfulness-oriented friends, and laughter from the cheery ones. While I seem to have many support systems in place, it was important for me to use the support. Most of the time, that worked for me. But I came to a point shortly after my Mom's passing when I hit the proverbial wall. I shouldered the burdens for a long time - - seven years - - and for the most part, I kept up the pace.

But on a Friday afternoon, my world became a bit unglued. I came home from work early, thinking that maybe the headache I couldn't shake would be better with more fluids, a nap, and an ice pack on my forehead, a combination that always seemed to work. But by 4 p.m., I had no tricks left, and my blood pressure was climbing to dangerous levels. Dave and I debated about "what next", and we decided a trip to the local emergency room was in order. He could not stay with me due to COVID restrictions, so after the triage staff ruled out a heart attack, I proceeded to wait for additional tests and the opportunity to talk with a physician.

The very kind and young physician came to see me about midnight, apologizing for the wait, and indicated that the tests showed no signs of cardiac issues. He then asked: has something significant happened in the last few months? And, of course, there was the Mom Event. We talked a bit about delayed stress reactions, which were not new to me. I had episodes of hair loss about three months after Dave's brain cancer surgery which resolved when he was on the mend. I could think of other, similar delayed ways in which I responded to stress. I went home that night with fairly normal blood pressure and an appointment with my primary care the following Monday.

On Monday I had a telehealth visit with Dr. Faith, who knows both Dave and me and our situation. After some conversation, I was a blubbery mess. The crying was uncontrollable, and I was embarrassed. She said: you need to cry. When is the last time you cried before today? I could not remember. Oh sure, there had been moments of tearing up, but the deep wails of grief that come from within were something from long ago.

I thought about that a lot. I was so grateful for my support, so many friends and family members, and colleagues whom I knew truly cared.

They helped me work through my caregiving duties. They made sure I got out for a treat, a reprieve. But I needed to work on my own internal stuff, and that was facing loss. It was loss beyond Mom; it was loss of what had been and will be no more. I had denied loss for so long, and I had not grieved its passing. Dr. Faith brought that fully home to me.

I sought support for this as I did for other needs in my cancer caregiving, except this time the aim was fully on my need to recognize and embrace the waves of emotion that wash over me. To sit with them, be with them, and not run them off to be productive or busy. My newest round table has members who have personally dug deep inside, find spaces to sit with me, suggest techniques or practices that guide me to better inner awareness of how I am truly doing.

This support has been difficult yet freeing. I am challenged to "be" and sit in the "now". Facing one's own "stuff" is not always easy. I have spent a lifetime of doing, thinking quickly, reacting. It is ingrained in me, and much of the time, it has served me well, until it hasn't. It is now a time to pause, reflect, and to sit with thoughts and not rush out on them to other things. And it was those at the round tables that brought me to this realization.

Round tables have always been part of my life. There are no head chairs at these tables, and everyone comes and sits equally among others. Everyone contributes their unique gifts. And I learn from them as they may perhaps learn from me. We sit in the now together, fully present in our moment. Round tables are my lifelines.

# Obtaining Support

# By
# Charlie Shockey

Without question, Erie and my livrd as cancer patient and caregiver, respectively, would have been far more difficult if we had not been surrounded by an enormous outpouring of support from many different sources. Following her initial diagnosis of metastatic breast cancer in 1992, Erie experienced a devastating blow to every aspect of her life, which suddenly went from that of a well-adjusted and fulfilling role as a mother, wife, and social worker to that of a 39-year-old cancer patient facing a very real prospect of losing everything within a short period of time. The most difficult challenge was figuring out how best to continue to love and nurture our two young sons, ages 10 and 6 while knowing that she may not be around to guide and raise them as she had always expected. We were so very fortunate to have a network of family, friends, and medical advisers who all pitched in to try to soften the shock of cancer as much as possible. One lesson I learned from that experience was that an open and candid approach to confronting Erie's life with cancer helped to bring in so many people and resources into the process that we quickly realized that we were not alone in trying to stabilize and reorder our lives.

The immediate outpouring of love from our families, while certainly not surprising, made all the difference to us in getting through Erie's diagnosis and the initial stages of treatment and recuperation. Her family devoted all their attention to helping us navigate through the minefield of decisions required by the need to sort through the options for diagnosis, surgery, and chemotherapy. While I have no doubt that we would have managed to cope with the overwhelming plethora of difficult decisions, the benefit of having her parents, her brothers, and their wives all volunteer their time and efforts helped to reassure us that our decisions made sense. They helped us work with the medical staff at Fairfax Hospital to make sure we received all the information we needed to make informed choices at every stage.

In addition, we were blessed to have a close-knit group of friends in the Washington, D.C. area who extended their love and support for Erie. Three couples who were among our closest friends, then and now, got together and purchased a Sony Walkman CD-player and a set of CDs for Erie to listen to during the many hours when she was resting at home following her chemo treatments. They also gave her several colorful, carved Native American tokens for healing, placed in a small wicker basket that sat by her bed for weeks, months, and years, as a constant reminder that she was loved by so many people who valued her friendship and would do anything to help her survive her battle with cancer. Recently, when a former work colleague of mine shared the news that his own daughter had been diagnosed with breast cancer at age 34, I re-gifted one of those tokens, a small turquoise bear, to her. Erie was a big believer in "paying it forward" by doing acts of kindness for others, just as her friends had done for her, and I took pleasure in passing along this small gift of caring to a young woman and mother who faced the difficult path that Erie had traveled a generation earlier.

One source of support that exists in many communities is a cancer support group of patients who are facing similar difficulties. In the early days following her treatment, Erie learned of a breast cancer support group organized through Fairfax Hospital in Northern Virginia. This group was particularly valuable, I believe, because it enables the cancer patient to spend time with others and provide a setting for the patient herself to share all the emotions that only a patient can fully experience. While Erie certainly appreciated the love and support from me, her family, and our friends, none of us could really know what it feels like to know that a disease has invaded your body, taken over your life, and threatened your very existence. Erie went to weekly or monthly meetings with this support group for the first year of her life as a cancer patient. She met several women who became life-long friends. At the same time, the group membership frequently changed, partly due to everyone's preferences and, sadly, due to the loss of several of the women who, over time, succumbed to the disease. This latter reality was a constant reminder that the struggle against cancer for all these women was a difficult and, at times, unsuccessful battle.

One other source of support for Erie was the medical community itself. Because she was so open and engaged with her doctors, nurses, and other caregivers, often challenging them, and frequently amusing them with her candid remarks, she received a great deal of helpful information and feedback that helped her to cope with life as a cancer patient. She formed a particularly close bond with her oncologist in Fairfax, Dr. Nicholas Robert, whom she continued to consult for eight years before we moved to California. Dr. Robert, along with his colleagues, was consistently open and candid about Erie's situation. He recommended the cocktail of high-dose chemotherapy that, while horrible to experience, ended up giving Erie a new lease on life. They provided the hope that she would have many more years not only to survive, but also to raise our sons and continue her career as a school social worker, which gave her tremendous pleasure. Following the chemo treatments, Dr. Robert prescribed tamoxifen, which Erie took for the recommended five-year regimen, then continued to take for several years thereafter. When Erie pressed Dr. Robert for advice on what she could do to reduce the possibility that the cancer would recur, he said only two words. "Don't smoke." That advice struck me, and I continue to share it with others. Erie had smoked as a teenager and into her 20s. When we started dating, I made it clear that she would have to quit smoking if we were to get involved romantically. She gamely complied, although she struggled periodically, especially on social occasions when she would spend an evening with her former smoking companions. She sheepishly confessed to me, on occasion, that she had "cheated," but she took Dr. Robert's words to heart and never smoked again. At least not tobacco!

All of Erie's wonderful support systems in suburban Northern Virginia, which had been in place for eight years, were in for a radical shakeup. Following something of a mid-life career crisis of my own when I turned 50, 1 proposed that we move from northern Virginia to Sacramento, California, as I arranged for a job transfer within the U.S. Department of Justice.

After an initial period of uncertainty and a series of family discussions, she agreed, and we made the move in January 2001. For me, I very much relished a change of pace after 28 years in the Washington, D.C. area. For her, however, this meant not only leaving behind her close network of friends, but also her career and work colleagues. Perhaps most significantly, the move also meant leaving behind the wonderful medical team that had enabled her to overcome the initial bout with breast cancer and move back into life with a renewed appreciation. By then, our boys were older and had weathered the trauma of watching their mom suffer through the initial years of cancer treatment and recuperation. Nate was heading off to college in California, and Dave, while more than a little reluctant to leave his comfortable life as an eighth grader in Fairfax, grudgingly came along to an entirely new life and community in Sacramento. The first year was particularly difficult for Erie. While we adapted quickly to the great weather in California and enjoyed exploring the State's many natural wonders, Erie discovered that it was more difficult to make connections in a new city, especially now that the boys were older, and we didn't have the benefit of our school and community as a source for engaging with other parents and families. One benefit of the move was that we were able to spend more time with her brother Aton and his wife Norma, with whom we were quite close.

After that first year, Erie began to find her footing. She became a social worker for a job readiness program in downtown Sacramento, working with women who were experiencing homelessness and who, almost always, were victims of every form of abuse imaginable. This work was unbelievably challenging and often frustrating, yet it gave Erie a real sense of purpose and meaning in her own life, as she could use her many skills to help these women find shelter, protect their children, seek out treatment programs, and, in many cases, go back to school or find employment. Over the next decade, as we eventually developed a new network of friends in Sacramento, Erie's work at the Women's Empowerment Program really provided a new and different kind of social support system for her. She dedicated herself to helping hundreds of women and their families as they struggled with the challenges of poverty, abuse, and their physical, mental, and emotional health. During this time, Erie's cancer had been in remission to the point where she rarely spoke of it. She had established new connections with doctors in Sacramento but expressed little concern about cancer as an ever-present cloud, the way it had for the first decade after her treatment. Life, in many respects, had returned to a new normal, one that enabled our entire family to prosper and enjoy life once again.

By 2012, Erie found herself frequently more tired, often experiencing pain in her lower back and hips. After acknowledging that the constant demands of work were contributing to her physical and emotional health and well-being, she decided to retire from her job shortly before she turned 60. By then, both boys were "fully launched," pursuing their careers in New York and Sacramento, respectively, and meeting the women whom they would marry. We enjoyed a series of memorable family vacations, always fully documented by Erie's wonderful photographs. Following a trip to Seattle in November 2012 to attend the wedding of her closest friend's daughter, Erie was overcome with exhaustion and severe pain in her hips and lower back, to the point where she struggled to walk through the airport on our return home. She promptly scheduled an appointment with her primary care doctor. Her assessment and expectation were that the pain was associated with an old injury in her thigh. I was busy at work on a new case on the day of her appointment, so a friend accompanied her to the doctor.

"Mom has cancer," our son Dave sobbed into the telephone from his office on December 10, 2012. He called me around 11:30 that morning, just as I had wrapped up a lengthy conference call on my new court case. My heart stopped, and I was speechless for a few seconds, but quickly regained my composure. Dave, then 25 and just starting his career as a financial auditor for the State, had just spoken to her on the phone. Her doctor had received the test results and give Erie the news that she always had feared, but never was prepared to hear. Dave and I both left work and drove home. Erie was in shock and devastated. We all were. Exactly 20 years after the initial diagnosis, her breast cancer had returned, this time as Stage Four metastatic cancer that spread through her body and appeared in the bones of her right thigh, hips, and lower back. The smooth flight pattern of our lives in recent years had just hit major turbulence, and it felt like a crash was imminent. Once again, cancer would dominate our lives and require me to resume my role as an active caregiver and head of Erie's support team.

We took a day to compose ourselves and to call Nate in New York with the bad news before we reached out to our support network of family and friends. The primary care doctor's assessment was direct and bleak. With a recurrence of Stage Four metastatic breast cancer, the prognosis was...terminal. Stated simply, Erie and I knew from that day that she would die. With the benefit of our prior experience, we knew enough to reach out to several of the leading cancer clinics around the country, rather than simply accepting the initial diagnosis. We sent the pathology report to the Fred Hutchinson Cancer Research Center in Seattle, the M.D. Anderson Cancer Center in Houston, the University of California, San Francisco (UCSF) Helen Diller Family Comprehensive Cancer Center in San Francisco, and the University of California, Davis (UCD) Cancer Center in Sacramento, among others.

The response from all the doctors with whom we spoke was unanimous and consistent. Erie's condition was terminal. Having been blessed with twenty more years than she initially had expected back in 1992 with having had the benefit of seeing our two sons grow up, mature, and find their own paths as young adults in their late 20s, Erie was far more philosophical and accepting of the terrible hand that she had been dealt. One lesson we both drew from having the recurrence occur later in our lives was that we both were more at peace with Erie's fate, now that we knew our sons and I could handle the sad news with a far greater sense of maturity. And yet, still...cancer sucks. Erie screamed it and cursed and cried along with me for several nights. Then, inevitably, we realized that life does, indeed, go on. And so must we. The biggest questions were how long she could expect to live and what quality of life she could be prepared to face.

At this point, while we continued to enjoy a profound outpouring of love and support from family and friends, our principal support group really consisted of the wonderful medical team that went to bat for Erie and helped her (and me) through the next four years. Following the recommendations of her new medical team, Erie first underwent radiation to alleviate the most immediate and pronounced pain in her back, hip, and thigh. Early in the process, while still trying to determine the best course of treatment, we arranged a consultation with Dr. Hope Rugo at UCSF. By all accounts, Dr. Rugo was among the leading breast cancer specialists in the nation. Erie, in her inimitable style, called her the "West Coast Boob Guru." We copied the several hundreds of pages of diagnostic pages that we had accumulated and drove to San Francisco for the day. Dr. Rugo spent close to three hours going over the reports with us and discussing Erie's situation. She concurred with the course of action outlined by Dr. Helen Chew at the UCD Cancer Center and agreed that it made the most sense for Dr. Chew to serve as the primary oncologist in charge of her care. Happily, we never sensed any personal rivalry or disconnect within the medical team. Their uniform concern was to care for Erie in every way possible. And, when pressed repeatedly by Erie as to how long she might expect to live, Dr. Chew emphasized that she could expect to live for some time, obviously with no guarantees. While the end result - death - now was clear, the focus of her medical care would be on how to maximize the quality of life, rather than focusing on the length of time expected to be available. This advice was essential for us to understand because we were faced with some pretty significant choices in terms of how best to spend our remaining time together.

From March 2013 through July 2016, Erie went through a series of hormonal treatments, then, when those treatments declined in efficacy, a series of chemotherapy treatments, all overseen by Dr. Chew at UCD. At each stage, Erie would undergo periodic PET scans to follow the status of the tumors. As Dr. Chew explained, recurrent breast cancer most often lodges in the bones or in soft tissue organs, including the liver, lungs, heart, or brain. While the bone impacts are painful, they tend not to be life-threatening, as would be the case when the cancer would attack the organs. Fortunately, which hardly seems like the right word, Erie's tumors were largely confined to the bones for the next several years.

Throughout the three years of active treatment regimens, before Erie opted to enter hospice care, the support provided by the UCD team of doctors, nurses, other medical staff, and everyone at the cancer center was extraordinary. Through their care and support, we had secured a new lease on life, albeit short-term, that would extend for more than four years. This new lease would provide us with the time needed to re-direct our lives to what mattered most, our family, our friends, and, of course, each other.

# Circling Wagons

## By
## Cindy Bowden

Randall and I were always private people. We depended mostly upon each other for 24 years. My cousin Tammy made the observation that I don't reach out for support and for the most part, neither did Randall. My support system was very different for Randall's two diagnoses. In 2016, we'd been living in Corpus Christi for six years and had a small network of close friends and colleagues. My mom, stepdad, youngest sister Deidre, and nephew Sebastian, lived the closest, at 370 miles away, east of Dallas. The rest of our family lived out of state. I had my friends, from teaching in the community and Randall had friends from TAMUCC and competing in triathlons. I treasured the ladies I worked with at Windsor Park Elementary. When I told them about Randall's diagnosis, my friend Ruthann took me straight to the Blessed Sacrament Convent and we wrote our intentions to give to the Sisters; mine of course being, "Please let Randall beat the cancer." She brought my friends together for a prayer group, checked on me weekly, if not daily, and wrote notes of encouragement to me and to Randall. My friend Renee was just as supportive. She'd ask me to meet for coffee and would simply listen. I know that secretly she was trying to get me out of the house and give me a little sunshine, and it worked. I'm so very grateful to them both, and to all of my friends for their support during that time. Colleagues from TAMUCC were there for Randall and me every step of the way. Kami would check in on Randall both personally and professionally. Randall took comfort in support from two of his fellow triathletes, Allen and Freddy. I'm so thankful for these three men. Along with our families, they boosted Randall's morale and helped give him the strength he needed to live through that fourth and final week of chemotherapy.

Our families have been a constant: supporting us both throughout the last 5 ½ years. My mom was born to be a wife and mother. She tells us that is all she ever wanted to do. However, she's so much more than that. She's a life-long learner and as a single mom, she went back to school at age 39 to earn her bachelor's and master's degrees in special education. She has been a positive role model for her children. The four of us have watched in awe as she worked tirelessly; first, to earn her degrees while working part time and raising a family, and then by teaching and supporting her students in the classroom. She's a mentor, and I can go to her with any question, or any situation and she will listen and guide me. Mom supported us both throughout the 5 ½-year rollercoaster ride of cancer. When Randall and I met in Denver in 1997, my family welcomed Randall with open arms. In fact, he and I used to joke that Randall became the new "favorite." Not only did my mom have to endure her daughter going through the difficulties of being a cancer caregiver, but she also watched as her son-in-law, (second son) battled and suffered. Our phone conversations saved my sanity and kept me grounded more than she will ever know.

The second time Randall was diagnosed with stage four cancer, in August of 2018, we had only lived in Granbury, Texas for a year. Randall was working for Tarleton State University, and I had just been hired as a kindergarten teacher in a neighboring town the day before Randall's diagnosis. He suggested I work during this cancer battle, if nothing else, to keep my mind occupied. I was teaching at a new school in a neighboring community where I knew no one.

Randall started his second cancer battle right after receiving his diagnosis and drove by himself to Houston each week to receive immunotherapy treatment. He would drive five hours, have the one to two-hour treatment and/or blood work, and drive back home five hours; all in one day. I only went one time that fall; when he was biopsied and needed family to drive him to and from the procedure. I was a wreck for those five months, imagining him falling asleep at the wheel or involved in a car accident. He was working 50+ hours a week while battling cancer by driving back and forth to MDA in

Houston from Granbury. I couldn't fully focus on my students, worrying about Randall driving solo to and from Houston, and on the occasions when I did go with him, I fretted about my class. I resigned my teaching position half way through the year. Only for my family, would I resign a teaching position mid-year. I was upset about leaving, the parents were upset I was leaving, and when the students were told, they were upset too. I think back and am so thankful to my principal, Joel, for understanding that I wanted and needed to be there with and for Randall.

Over the course of two and a half years, we drove thousands of miles, stayed in hotels hundreds of days, and flew more than 100 hours to fight cancer. The Galleria Drury Inn in Houston became a home away from home. Nearly all of Randall's cancer treatment was outpatient which meant finding lodging near MD Anderson. The managers and employees at the Drury Inn were so supportive and knew us by name. It was difficult enough to go through cancer in the comfort of your own home, let alone with strangers in a different city. The community at the Drury made the experience as tolerable and as comfortable as it could be.

The staff at MDA was fabulous and very supportive. I knew that when Randall did travel alone, he was in good hands there. From the phlebotomists to the oncologists, Randall received excellent care. We were so grateful that he had access to these medical professionals. We would marvel at the fact that out of all the states, we just happened to be living in Texas when Randall was diagnosed only 270 miles away from MD Anderson, one of the top two hospitals for cancer treatment in the country.

I needed to go back to work and was hired as a paraprofessional in Granbury ISD. The support I've received from friends and colleagues in this community has helped me through this second cancer experience. I believe this is the reason we landed in Granbury, the last of our seven moves. After teaching nine years in Texas, I'd saved 45 personal days. I used every one of these days and the 20 I earned while working in GISD to fight cancer alongside my husband. Upon being hired, I informed my principal that Randall was a cancer survivor and that the immunotherapy treatments were stopping the metastatic melanoma from spreading. My principal at the time, Stacie, was extremely compassionate and supportive. She did not have to approve a total of 65 days off over the course of my two years as a paraprofessional, but she did so every time I made a request. When Stacie approved my requests for days off, she did it with a word of encouragement, a hug, a smile, and most often, all of the above. When I told her in the winter of 2021 that I wanted, applied for, and would need a teaching position for the next school year, she hugged me and said, "Understood."

# SUPPORT

## By
## Diane Linick

Support during a cancer journey comes in many forms. My sister had and greatly welcomed and appreciated her immediate family and dear friends as her team of caregivers. I wanted to also help her husband, son, and daughter, and my parents through this unthinkable journey. My mother and I formed a special bond caring for Ellen and I was awed by my mother's strength. We freely shared with one another how we were feeling throughout the course (and after) of Ellen's illness. I knew I could count on my husband's and kids' love of Ellen and their support as well. They understood that I needed to "be there."

I am also forever grateful for Ellen's Hospice nurse. She was there for Ellen's difficult final month and modeled what compassionate care looks like. Maureen was there for everyone's well-being during the most stressful time of our family's life, especially for Ellen's loving husband and children. I personally mention Ellen's nurse because I credit her gracious support and experience through which I learned much about the role of being a cancer caregiver. So as not to take her attention away from Ellen, Maureen and I developed a routine of walking out to her car together and debriefing about Ellen's present condition and her immediate needs plus the emotional and physical changes that may occur next. In 2004 my mother and I shared being my father's caregivers after his leukemia diagnosis. I was working full time, but my mother had cut back her hours. With his medical history and age, the doctors and my parents agreed that his treatment was going to be transfusions to help with his fatigue. This along with his Parkinson's disease issues added to his falls and further diminished his quality of life. Each week I would take my parents to the hospital for his treatment until they no longer helped him.

Shortly thereafter my dad stopped the treatments and Hospice was called. Fortunately, I was able to reflect on what I had learned about support from my sister's Hospice nurse and in turn be of help to them.

"Being there" for each other definitely describes the support system my husband and I embraced in life and certainly during his cancer journey. Our kids were there for David and me in every way. We were so grateful for their visits, especially when they brought our young grandchildren. Everyone needs to smile, and kids are the best medicine!

We had wonderful and understanding friends and upon hearing of David's cancer diagnosis they immediately called to offer their support and help with whatever David and I needed. David was still processing how quickly his life had changed and wasn't comfortable with me sharing his medical information. Due to our mutual belief in privacy, I totally agreed. He didn't want people offering him sympathy or false hope. Therefore, we worked out a plan whereby a few of our closest friends would relay the information that David was willing to share with our other friends and work contacts. This enabled me to use my time at school with my coworkers each day more efficiently (less socializing and giving me space to focus on work). I knew they were aware and understood. My friend and reading specialist mentor was gracious about substituting for me when I took leave to be with David. I knew my students would be in good hands. Having her was great support for me and the students as well.

Knowing David's comfort level, I supported and carried out his decisions relating to when and where he felt comfortable being with others. I honored and respected his wishes, yet I felt badly about turning away their sincere support. They wanted to talk, visit, and cook for us. I did keep David informed of their gestures and assured them we were very appreciative of their kindness. As time went on, I realized that in our own ways we needed more than just close family for support.

In truth, I feel David and I could have benefited from their help literally and emotionally. David's closest running friend called him for a run one day soon after David told him about his diagnosis. At dinner that night David, based on his friend's experience and encouragement, asked if I would go with him to speak with someone at a cancer support center, The Gathering Place. His friend had gone there the previous year for counseling after losing his wife. He wished he and his wife had known about The Gathering Place at the beginning of their journey. I had heard wonderful reviews about The Gathering Place, a not-for-profit organization that provides the patients, their spouses, children, parents, and siblings of cancer patients a wide variety of programs to meet their needs socially, emotionally, and physically within their facility. Counseling was also available to their caregivers as a special support when needed. I was not sure if David could even entertain the idea at this time during his illness. He was already overwhelmed with the enormity of being a cancer patient. After his initial tests and procedures were scheduled and done I, myself, was planning to suggest The Gathering Place as a resource for us. Ironically, (and fortuitously), his friend had the same idea about the same place! I was thrilled that it came from a trusted friend who had already been there and found it helpful to his family! This was a gift to David that he immediately wanted to share with me to help us navigate his cancer travels. We both agreed we could benefit from professional guidance and encouragement at this time. David met with one of the counselors alone for the first visit. They had me join the next two appointments. David was grateful to have his pressing questions and concerns addressed. The counselor knew he felt relief that he could and should have a voice in his treatment plan. He would find he was still "himself." Those meetings were what he needed. Even though I only went a few times during the journey, it was comforting to know that I had her as a contact at any point when I might need her insight. Most meaningful to us was that she assured us that it was in our nature to support each other and that we always would.

David was extremely close to his family, even though his two older sisters over the years had married and moved to Florida and raised their families there. His parents also moved from Ohio to Florida as they wanted to be closer to their daughters. David's sisters and my family in town immediately began helping our cause by researching for hospitals known for studying new treatments for melanoma.

They helped us by making appointments for interviews with the specialists and gathering David's dermatologist's notes, other test results and comments. David and I were busy making appointments for consultations with local doctors working with melanoma patients. At the same time, we spent hours reading and getting familiar with skin cancer. Everyone we and our family spoke to concluded that staying in Cleveland would be their recommendation for David's care. After all, we have two top hospitals that were both involved with research and new cancer trials. Family would be nearby, and David could work at home and rest when necessary. As it turned out, staying in Cleveland was to our advantage in all ways.

David was at The Cleveland Clinic for most of his care. He trusted and had an excellent relationship with his lead doctor at the Clinic. The doctor's demeanor was exactly what David could respond to. He was calm, serious, and honest with him each visit. This gave him complete confidence in his ever-changing care plan. When he needed another trial and his hospital wasn't able to run it, as we had hoped, University Hospital had recently set up the kind of trial that our doctor recommended. David needed to spend a few days each week in the intensive care unit to receive this medication. The doctors from both of our hospital teams met weekly to monitor David's care. I did not have to be the one passing information between his two doctors. We were amazed at their support and appreciated how well-informed they kept us, often hourly. Nurses were monitoring him around the clock as there was a risk for a cardiac event at any time. I was there and so appreciated the respect and honesty the nurses shared with me. As unbelievably busy as they were, they constantly inquired how I was doing. Without their support, I would have been standing there alone frightened from listening to and watching machines and alarms. We spoke to one of his doctors after each treatment cycle. I was thankful for the accommodations that allowed me to sleep overnight. We assured David that security would escort me from the ICU to a small, locked meeting room with a couch. Several times I was called from the ICU and was back at his side within minutes.

As David knew I was "there" for him, he especially loved and appreciated the support from our children. Brian, our son, would often stop by at the hospital with a milkshake or other treat for David and meals for us. Amy, our daughter, and I were communicating multiple times a day, even trying to FaceTime. Amy lives in Michigan and helped me by informing our extended family through texts and calls about what was happening while David was in the ICU. That allowed me to be solely focused on David without walking away from the ICU to update others. During the second cycle, they began lowering the dose, which was very upsetting. As all had feared, after several weekly cycles, David's liver function, kidneys, lungs, and heart couldn't tolerate anymore. He was running a fever so they sent him from the ICU to a room on the oncology floor. He was coughing and having trouble breathing. X-rays and scans were taken of his chest and pneumonia was evident and antibiotics were started immediately. He was weak and restless. (Fortunately, I was able to stay in his room that night.)

The next day David's lead hematologist-oncologist at The Clinic called to tell me that the two hospital's lead doctors agreed that David would not be able to continue with the trial. We went in to meet with our Clinic doctor three days later so that he could explain David's body's reaction to this trial and then inquired as to what David's questions and personal wishes were at that point. David asked about his prognosis, a question that was always on his mind since his melanoma Stage IV diagnosis. The doctor answered weeks. David then announced he was done, no more hospitals, trials, IVs, blood tests, or pain. His doctor recommended The Clinic's palliative care support or Hospice. David chose hospice and acknowledged that he now wanted to have family and closest friends visit or call. He hoped he had the energy to follow through on his plan. David, being the gentleman that he was, thanked his doctor for his support, empathy, and honesty throughout this most trying time of his life. In turn, his doctor reiterated that no one could have been braver and that he was honored to have been his guide through his cancer journey.

# A Caregiver Obtains Support

## By
## Sonja McCaughey

My role as a caregiver for Nikita was to pray for her, care for her 4-year-old brother, support my son with everything that he needed to accomplish as a father, husband, a soldier, and support my daughter-in-law while she stayed with Nikita. Within four months of Nikita's diagnosis, I would have my four-year-old grandson Levi living with me in Florida while his sister and mom were in Maryland and his father was moving their home from Germany to Florida.

My role as Grammie was to support my family in whatever way they needed. Before my grandson would come to the United States, he would live with his maternal aunt who lives in Belgium. The Army would need to change my son's deployment to return to the United States where Nikita's medical treatment would continue. The options for her care were California, Maryland, Texas, and Florida. Nikita's doctors were also military physicians, and they needed to support the family, execute orders to where my son's deployment would change, and find a medical facility that would care for Nikita's medical care. This takes time. I asked what I could do to help out. My son and daughter-in-law decided along with me that my grandson would come live with me until the family could all move to Florida. My daughter-in-law has distant family in Florida, and it would be closer for her mother to fly from South America to Florida when needed. The Army knew where we would continue Nikita's care and now it was up to them to find the medical facility. While those orders were being prepared, my grandson would come live with me for the next 8 months along with his dad. Since I have four dogs already living in my home, bringing another dog into an established pack of dogs was not an option. Support came for the family dog to be cared for by a family in Germany.

When I decided to retire from the Tampa Police Department in October of 2016, my house was under construction. My son moved into the guest room and my grandson's bedroom was in my living room. My son would be traveling to Germany by himself to pack up their home and have their belongings shipped to Florida. There were many calculated trips to get his son, and the dog, continue working as a soldier, and be with his daughter. Military life is hard for everyone.

When I learned that Nikita had leukemia, I was attending Walden University working to earn my Ph.D. in law and public policy. In short order, I was dealing with a four-year-old little boy in the house who did not understand what was going on with his family and why he could not have his dog live with him. I made the decision to leave the university until my son's family was all together. I prayed that I would provide good support for my son and to provide awesome support for my grandson. He was confused and angry, but it was certainly understandable. I remember one night after we said our prayers that little boy told me "I love you Grammie;" my heart melted.

All of us were being pulled in different directions while we all tried to support each other in the battle against cancer. None of us knew what our future was going to look like and none of us were certain if we were doing the right thing at the right time for the right reasons to fight cancer. We were all over the place, literally in different parts of the world, to fight one cancer while supporting each other. The separation strained our family relations and at times we all wanted to scream and throw up our arms in frustration and assess blame for the battle with ALL that had been thrust on us and it would have been the right action because we were not together.

Nikita's mom decided social media would be a way to inform family and friends about the progress of Nikita's treatment. This brought support from friends and family that was geographically spread out all over the world. Short videos came in with words of encouragement, silly jokes, pictures of people that Nikita missed interacting with, and prayers. Every card Nikita received was taped on the walls of her room. A simple interaction of seeing people you cannot see because you are away from them, then being quarantined because of cancer, and missing your friends, social media provided a wonderful support system for Nikita and her friends and for the extended family.

I decided the best support that I could offer as Grammie was to embrace the moments of being there for my son's family and being a surrogate parent to my grandson. I learned about his favorite foods and his favorite cartoons. I learned his favorite songs that he wanted to hear when we took road trips. My grandson and I became friends. We made videos to send to Nikita about climbing tree stands and how to swing on a tire swing and pictures of whatever Levi thought his sister would want to see; he too offered support to his sister.

Even with the support of the military and the physicians who cared for Nikita we all felt very alone. I blame the great distance that separated us and the inability to give hugs and wipe away tears when needed. A one-way trip by car to visit Nikita was 1000 miles. Phone calls were just not enough to give adequate support; however, that's all we had. Air flights were expensive.

The time it took to prepare for a puppy sitter, time off from work, and then try to stay healthy so there was no possibility to contaminate an already sick little girl was stressful. It becomes easy to become isolated when you are trying to stay healthy. Cancer is not fair. Retiring from the police department was the best decision for me and my family to make although I lost my support system of friends and colleagues whom I had worked with for a very long time. When I retired from TPD, I moved two hours north from where I worked for 20 years and four months. Much of my time at the agency was working in a major crime unit and most of my colleagues were retiring about the same time as I was. My friends were going off in different directions in their retirement and support from them came in phone calls. I did not expect support from my friends because it was a battle against cancer in a child they did not know. It is difficult to hear that a child has cancer. When Nikita was diagnosed with leukemia in August 2016, I had just celebrated my twentieth year with the police force in July and my daughter had graduated from college in May. Now one of my oldest babies needed my help and I made a significant decision for the benefit of me, Nikita and the rest of the family.

Leaving the agency was not a difficult decision to make. I had a great career and enjoyed the work that I did. Policing took me away from birthday celebrations, dinner plans, dance recitals, and other plans that had to be canceled. I do not miss being wakened and called out in the middle of the night and trying to explain to my family why someone's family appears to be more important than they are. The list of things that took me away from my family to serve the public is quite long. I still wake up at the sound of a bug having a hiccup. However now, being available to my family was my priority. I was fortunate to have financial support in place that would allow me to retire and support my family with anything they wanted or needed.

I look back from the time my son called me. I wished I had offered support differently. They say during times of diversity we learn more about people. I knew from the beginning what my role was as mom and Grammie and I wished I had been more patient, more loving, and less angry with cancer and the unknown future. When Nikita was 15, I asked her if she felt she was supported through this difficult time in her life. Without hesitation she said yes and that everyone supported her the best way they could. She did not name any one person as being better than anyone else. After she gave her answer, I realized she was right. We all supported her the best we could. She is alive and is healthy and tomorrow is looking really good for her.

As for support for me, I am a private person. Those that knew about Nikita's cancer would ask about her and they still do today. It warms my heart when people ask about how she is doing. It is these very same people that have unknowingly offered support when I am able to talk about her and her journey. I used to be a hospice volunteer and the people that I have been with when their time had come taught me how support was important not only for those who were dying but as well as for those who cared for them. Having a keen sense of self-awareness while taking care of someone whom you know is very sick or may die helps you to make sure you take care of yourself. It helps in understanding the disease and probability of life or when death will happen to each person in hospice; however, caregivers need to take time to heal themselves for our process of caregiving.

I have healed from hearing about Nikita's cancer. It took many prayers and probably more tears than prayers to get out the confusion of how Nikita ended up with cancer, the hurt I caused when I lost my patience, and the anger of what cancer does to not only the person who had the cancer but for all of us who watched the treatment. I have healed knowing that she will be okay. I have accepted that life is short and the best way to heal from a devastation called cancer is to live life. I have learned that even though I was Grammie through this, faults, and all, I was helpful. Talking to my family and friends has always been helpful and without communication with them and God, healing has been easy.

# Determining A Treatment Strategy

## By
## Elizabeth Hapner

Diagnosis is only the first step in a long process. Coming to terms with a potentially catastrophic diagnosis was a lengthy process but it had to be initially accepted very quickly in order to get on with the treatment protocol required to extend his life. Kyle and I were both people of tremendous faith and we relied on that faith to get through the arduous process of treatment. Were it not for our firm belief that he would be going to a better place if he did not survive, and that we would be reunited someday, I do not know how either of us would have dealt with the harsh reality of his diagnosis.

Well prior to his diagnosis, Kyle's pain level was generally a 7 or 8 on a scale of 10. In August 2017, we took a wonderful trip to South Africa. One day Kyle was not up to going on our safari. Given his huge love of animals, and the fantasy nature of the trip, this was very concerning to me. Although he was placed on a significant amount of narcotic pain medication after his diagnosis, his pain never really subsided. Consequently, he remained in a physically diminished and mentally compromised state throughout the balance of his life. Managing his pain level became a key element of his treatment.

When we went to Moffitt for advice, and then treatment, we noticed that we never saw other patients in his age range. Given the statistics, this was surprising. Kyle was assigned a supportive care physician, who happened to be the department chair. Her assistance throughout his treatment was invaluable, even though he declined a number of the assistance options available to him. We were extremely fortunate to have Moffitt Cancer Center, one of the top ten national cancer centers, right here in Tampa. Treatment at Moffitt started with a series of additional screening, comprehensive testing, and scans. Our initial visit with his surgeon was very brief and not particularly informative. We then had to await the initial decision of the complex case team as to the course of treatment. This team, made up of his surgeon, oncologist and other experts, reviewed all of his scans and test results and decided whether surgery was an option. To say the wait was stressful would certainly be an understatement. Unfortunately, the news, when it arrived, was not what we wanted to hear but we would still be given hope as the team would re-evaluate the situation after a course of chemotherapy. We were determined to leave no stone unturned in our quest for a successful outcome but quickly learned that the treatment protocol postponed options such as immunotherapy until there was no other available treatment option.

While I secretly continued to wonder why this was happening to the center of my world, I began making the necessary changes to my law practice to permit me to be available for Kyle's treatments while supporting our needs financially. A reduction to my workload as a sole practitioner was required and a change in the focus of my practice to reduce the time spent in court. The local bench was very supportive, permitting me to postpone some hearings and to appear telephonically for others. The first hearing I had after Kyle's diagnosis actually took place with me on my cell phone as we walked through the hospital to the area where Kyle would have another colonoscopy. The connection from a hospital, with all of the computer and other equipment in use, was certainly less than ideal but the judge, a breast cancer survivor, made it work.

One of Kyle's initial questions related to preservation of sperm. He was just thirty years of age and very much wanted children if he survived and possibly even if he did not. After a frank discussion with his oncologist, he came to the difficult acknowledgment that it would not be fair to bring a child into the world when he very likely would not be there to parent that child. While the issue of sperm preservation was not one I had considered before he raised it, it  was also very painful for me to accept the reality that not only would I likely lose my beloved only child but also would never have any grandchildren. Strategizing a treatment plan was not something in which Kyle or I had much input. Nor were we given the level of information as to the actual process that I would have preferred. There was no scheduled number of chemotherapy treatments for Kyle. It was simply every other Friday for as long as it was having any positive effect. It was very difficult for me to walk past the bell that is rung each time a patient successfully completes chemotherapy, knowing that bell would never be rung for Kyle. Kyle never commented on it but you could tell it affected him each time it was rung for someone while we were there for his treatment.

Although treatment is different for each patient, my strong recommendation to any parent navigating this journey is that you find someone who has been down this path already and get as much information from that person as possible. If you cannot find a parent of a prior patient, find a spouse or other family member who is willing to give you the guidance you should have. Our experience was that while the treatment team gives you a lot of information, they do not think about the little details you would find helpful. We were fortunate to be given a corporate care representative because I was acquainted with Lee Moffitt and some of the other board members. She accompanied us on our first several visits to Moffitt for testing and treatment and answered questions by phone and email, but her focus was on the information related to the administration of the treatment and how to get around the large facility. Details such as how to read his test results on the website, how to get an Internet connection in the facility, hours of operation for the cafeteria and what to bring with you when you came for chemotherapy was not included in the information conveyed to us.

Everything possible was done to make Kyle feel comfortable and as positive as he could be throughout. The atmosphere overall was very hopeful, with musicians, support dogs, comfortable seating areas and other amenities to ease the process. Despite this, the sheer size of the facility and number of patients was rather intimidating. His oncologist's primary nurse was very upbeat and welcoming. Kyle's mantra, anytime he needed anything was "Call Bonnie" and later "Call Amanda" (nurse to his supportive care physician). Because Kyle was still able to work for the first few months of his treatment and to accommodate my work schedule as well, Kyle's chemotherapy sessions were scheduled for alternate Fridays. Kyle was sent home, late on Friday afternoons, with a chemotherapy pump, and we had to return to the main campus on Sundays to have it removed and more blood drawn. Initially, chemotherapy took place at the main campus, but Kyle did not like the hectic pace and large number of people at that chemotherapy center, complaining that it was "a bunch of old, sick people." There were three local locations for chemotherapy, each of which we tried for treatment. Sundays we always traveled to the main facility because it was the only one open then, but it was practically deserted by comparison to weekday visits so despite the greater distance, it was not a hardship.

The second treatment took place at another of the locations which was much more convenient in terms of parking and access, but Kyle again found it overwhelming in size and number of patients. A friend of mine had been undergoing breast cancer treatment and told me that the least crowded and geographically most convenient chemotherapy treatment center was one in central Tampa, by a mall. Scheduling time at that facility was much easier and Kyle much preferred the location, both in terms of the physical location and the physical plant itself. That change made a definite improvement in Kyle's mental attitude. As a parent, obtaining such information and making such seemingly insignificant adjustments is a minor task in exchange for a much greater level of comfort for your child.

Every patient handles the flow of information as to his condition and treatment differently. For example, Kyle often did not want to be in the room when his father or I asked certain questions as to his current status. Nor did he generally want to know his tumor markers. Kyle's focus was on maintaining the most positive attitude possible and ignorance of certain information assisted him in maintaining that focus. In order to remain hopeful, Kyle simply could not consider certain facts and to a large degree, was in denial as to just how serious his diagnosis was.

As a longtime "control freak," the idea of relinquishing any control over my course of treatment to others was unimaginable. Ultimately, Kyle made the major decisions, but he was not generally interested in making the small ones. He had always relied on me and chose to continue to do so in this instance. At other times, he would say "Mom, I'm dying of cancer so just let me do _____" whatever it was he had in mind at the time.

Actual chemotherapy sessions were a learning experience. First, Kyle had to have blood drawn. After the results were reviewed by his oncologist, there was a window of approximately two hours before his chemotherapy cocktail was readied by the lab. If we did not have an appointment with the oncologist in the interim period, we would generally go get breakfast.

Kyle needed as many calories as he could tolerate consuming, and we knew he would not have an appetite after chemotherapy. Generally, only one person was permitted to accompany Kyle to chemotherapy sessions, but they usually looked the other way when a second person arrived.

Chemotherapy facilities, and cancer facilities in general, are always cold. Cancer makes the patient much more susceptible to cold, so we learned immediately to have Kyle wear a hoodie and to bring his favorite blankets and extra socks. While I generally attempted to get some work done during his chemo, Kyle generally slept or watched television. A pair of good wireless earbuds I bought him proved to be a very useful purchase. Also of great use was a wireless hotspot, coupled with my VPN, since I found the Internet connection in the facilities to be less than consistently reliable.

Fatigue, pain, and neuropathy required that Kyle cease working by Labor Day, 2018. His job in logistics coordination at a freight logistics company not only required him to sit for many hours but also required his consistent availability. Taking advantage of COBRA, we maintained Kyle's health insurance. If at all possible, this is the preferable option for the first eighteen to twenty-four months.

Fortunately, Kyle only had one hospitalization after his initial diagnosis, just a month prior to his death. In the interim, he did have to make several trips to Moffitt Urgent Care. Unlike an emergency room, Moffitt Urgent Care required advance permission. Each time I would have to call, invariably on a weekend, describe the issue and await a return call telling me that a physician had approved his visit. An urgent care visit was also required while we were at M.D. Anderson in Houston but that visit was initiated by the physician who had seen a blood clot on Kyle's scan. For his later visits, an ambulance service also had to be arranged.

The day-to-day dynamics of life with a cancer patient could be trying. Appointments at Moffitt tended to be scheduled for early in the morning so that we could get blood work done, see his oncologist and have time left to complete treatment that day. Invariably, I would be up and ready to go and Kyle would not be. Because of his condition, it took time for him to go to the bathroom and get ready for the day took longer because his pain made him move more slowly. Adjusting to this reality was hard for me. "Chemo brain" was also a reality. Organization and double-checking became key to ensuring that things did not get missed or left behind. "Not sweating the small stuff" became a necessary motto.

Immunotherapy brought a whole new learning process, at a new location and with a whole new set of healthcare providers, aside from his oncologist. All immunotherapy treatments were done at the main campus. After checking in, Kyle would have blood drawn within that area as opposed to the main lab. We would wait for an hour or so while his oncologist and other treatment team members received and reviewed the results. The infusion would be formulated and then

Kyle would begin his treatment. This was a heart-wrenching process because Kyle did not react well to the immunotherapy treatments. Our hopes for an extended life expectancy were resting solely on this new form of treatment which had shown such promising results.

# Chapter 3:

# Hope

# Seeing the Stars

## By
## Linda W. Devine

The verbal affirmation of Dave's cancer diagnosis sent me to a frozen place. Before driving to Moffitt Cancer Center for the first meeting with Dr. Tan, we rehearsed our responses, given the evidence that we had. We brainstormed our questions and determined that I would be the questioner. My notebook and pen were ready. We prepared for the worst, but we are hopeful people. But even for one of my temperaments, which has been called "Pollyanna" at times, officially receiving the diagnosis sent me to a dark and cold place emotionally. I asked the questions, jotted down notes, and otherwise performed with robotic precision, all on plan. Dave did not speak, also our plan, but was uncharacteristically immoveable, a gray concrete statue of himself.

The world had shifted; I was off kilter, soldiering on through the appointment. But somehow, hope would rise. Even as we took the car ride back to what would be our new life with cancer, we were trying to find bright spaces, signs of what could be. Our immediate attention was on our three adult children and our mothers and how we would convey the news. The cancer would re-shape their lives, too. And so, we intentionally chose to see the situation as a challenge through which we would persevere, almost low-balling the effect it would have on how we lived. I often think of my dear friend Viva who told me about one of her techniques for mentally handling stress. She thinks of her brain as a large room with many shelves. (We agreed we both have large brain rooms as we have lived long and have lots of information stored there!) On those shelves sit boxes, each labeled with a part of her life. When a stressful situation arises, she takes that box down from the shelf, gives the contents its time. She then puts the contents back in the box, lid affixed, and places the box back on the shelf for another day. Cancer would have its box in our life, but it would not be the biggest box nor would it be a central feature of our existence.

Hope has emanated from many places and experiences over my life. My faith journey is a profound source of hope, including the formalized teachings of my Catholic upbringing, the Protestant communities to which I now belong, and the acceptance of eastern thought through meditation practice. While I used to think of these traditions as discrete concepts, experience is showing me that there is a fluidity of thought, perhaps universal truth, that runs across the boundaries that we humans have set.

Each of these traditions calls for introspection and a concomitant search for something wider or higher than this earthly realm. When hope dissipates, and darkness creeps back into my life, as it is wanting to do, I reach for the comfort of these belief systems. They are now my mental muscle memory, and I instinctively move to prayer and meditation, whether it is in response to sadness, joy, discomfort, or indecision.

Some have suggested that a set time and place for prayer and meditation is optimal. While this sounds nice and tidy to me as a creature of habit and a planner by profession, caregiving sometimes does not afford the luxury of a "set time and place". Cancer is not on a schedule, and neither are the needs of those that it afflicts. Sometimes it was preparing food or dispensing pills that were not on "the schedule" or tending to a wound or cleaning garments. Sometimes it was dealing with nausea or pain.

Linens may need changing at inopportune times, or it may be a consult with medical personnel or a non-routine appointment, or a run to the pharmacy. Professional caregivers, as wonderful as they can be (and ours were), have their own lives and responsibilities, and pivoting to cover their duties when they are unavailable is to be expected. So, the scheduling of prayer and meditation were not possible, as I learned. Sunday church services, which I attended regularly, were now hit or miss, as were other scheduled, reflective activities. I found, however, something better. Prayer and meditation need not wait for the grand moment of the day or evening to be beneficial. They became part of my routines. I take comfort in the everyday: folding clothing, washing dishes, vacuuming, and other seemingly uninspiring household tasks. My home became my temple, my actions my petitions. I found my solace and hope in focusing on the necessary activities of daily living. When I wake up, I think about the hymn Make Me A Blessing (for someone today), ironically using a western song to set an eastern intention for the day. As I prepped a meal, I thought about the food and the people who made it possible to be in my kitchen and those that created the kitchen tools and recipes. While keeping an eye on my loved ones, rocking in my chair with a cup of tea, I reflected on the moment and the beyond. I spoke to what I believe to be my extended choir of the faithful, wherever they may be. I repeated the ancient prayers and mantras. And I asked the Universe to Be Thou My Vision, an Irish hymn that implores a greater power to guide and provide light in the darkness. And it is through these acts, woven into my day, that I found signs of hope. It might be the effects of medicine and nutrition or physical therapy, strengthening the bodies of those challenged. In the book of Psalms, the writer David says that "I am fearfully and wonderfully made". Our bodies are gloriously complicated. As I look back on photos of my Dave when we did not know he had cancer and compare them to images of today, the work of the medicine, nutrition, and physical activity are evident. And I saw the same in my Mom, who had renal failure, C. difficile, along with other ailments. Once she had months of good food and an effective medicine program, along with physical and occupational therapies, she reemerged from her shrunken, feeble state and lived well past what was expected in a quality way that she enjoyed.

My routine tasks of preparing food, ensuring medicine doses were taken and bodies were moving, were part of my hope routine, reinforced by what I witnessed. And hope shows itself in other ways, and I learned that I needed to be open and attentive. When I am open to what the Universe is telling me, I see the manifestations of hope. I see that when I did not think there was a chance, life will continue, just perhaps not in the form that I had imagined. I am an avid gardener, and I love getting into the weeds and the dirt, even on the hottest Florida days. I feel alive with the burning sun and the resultant sweating, creating a human-inspired order out of plants that grow like crazy here ten months of the year. I sit in the cool shade of the patio or maybe under the sycamore tree, pondering the miracle of nature. And, I have learned, the weeds are the ultimate sign of hope. No matter how hard I try to keep the weeds at bay, they always seem to reappear in large and small ways. Small flowers bud in the concrete cracks, vines meander through the pine mulch, and shoots climb the bricks. Leaves flutter through the driveway, the tabebuia tree creates seasons of a lovely "mess" with its pods and effusive pink flowers, needing a near daily clean-up. And these plants have companions – ants, snakes, raccoons, squirrels, woodpeckers, birds – they come along for the ride.

Despite my best efforts, hope springs eternal in the flora and fauna. So why should it not be in our human realm? And hope abides with relationships, both human and animal. During dark moments, a phone call from a friend can make a difference. My friendship circles have lifted me in many ways, some of which I am sure I will never know. From phone calls to squirreling me away for a glass of wine or a hot meal, it has made all the difference in rebalancing and re-kindling hope.

My friend Winnie, a much better plant tender than me, will ferry us to the nearest orchid show or to the University of South Florida Botanical Gardens, where I can lose myself in the divine sights and smells of the earth and its plants. Or Jan and
Julia, for whom sharing many evenings has produced laughter and sports talk and eating fests. It was and is these friends and untold other guardian angels that come alongside and walk a piece of my path with me. They are my human respite heroes, and they have a way of sharing the wider world, a hopeful world. And hope is in my furry friends, too. Phoebe Lisa and Cheese Pizza Marie (yes, those are their names) are major partners in experiencing hope. In the dark

moments, these critters greeted me with unbridled joy. They forced me to play and snuggle, even when I was not particularly in the mood. They are my walking partners, sometimes multiple times during a day, when I needed fresh air and a short break before resuming care tasks. And, dogs live in the moment, like my faith traditions ask me to do.

We worry about yesterday and tomorrow, and when we do this; we give up time in our present. Phoebes and Pizza always return me to the "now". Time has no hold on them – they enjoy the sunshine, nap when they need to, and delight in those around them. Having them in our home has been a joy, not only for me but in particular for Mom, for whom Pizza kept guard until she transitioned. While my journey has been a relatively happy one, darkness periodically invades my space. Not all moments are joyous; some are less so. It is often in the middle of the night that I experience a dark internal emotional state, poignantly matching my surroundings. But pulling away from yesterday and not awfulizing tomorrow are lessons that I have learned along this caregiver path. The center of those lessons was the intended outcome of hope. The faith traditions, actions, and friends that I have cultivated over a lifetime are my support systems that imbue hope in me, and without this hope, I cannot imagine life.

What would a life look like without hope? Even those who have suffered greatly spoke of hope. Anne Frank, in her diary, wrote that "I don't think of all the misery, but of the beauty that still remains." Finding hope in the everyday dispels the darkness even for the moment. While my lived experience is unlike Anne Frank's, I am in receipt of the purity of her words, the thoughts of a young girl in the midst of awfulness, still looking to the beauty that exists beyond misery. And therefore, I choose to hope. The antithesis of that choice would be unbearable. And the darkness that I first felt on the day of diagnosis is a bit less frightening now. Dr. Martin Luther King, Jr., in his last speech, said "But I know, somehow, that only when it is dark enough can you see the stars". I find this sentiment to be exceedingly comforting, as time spent feeling alone and in the dark, both externally and internally, can be overwhelming. Caregivers like me sometimes think that we are alone in the universe, but we are not. And Dr. King says that we can use that darkness to see beauty. I remember my mother-in-law telling the grandkids that when they saw the moon and the stars each night, that she would be there, too, watching them from wherever she was in the world or beyond. I like to think that we all find solace in a starry night, arms linked, whether here or in the greater Universe, using the darkness to make the connections even more bright.

# Hope And A Roller Coaster Life

## By
## Charlie Shockey

Life with cancer is a roller coaster, figuratively and, in our case, literally, as well. Like a roller coaster, we experienced so many heart-stopping drops in emotion, each followed, in time, with a rise in hope as we mounted up the next hill. From the time of my wife Erie's initial diagnosis of metastatic breast cancer in 1992, through her final days in 2017, she experienced the full range of human emotions, many times over, sometimes in the same hour or day. In my role as her primary caregiver for that quarter century, I also experienced the highs and lows with her, although I was always conscious of the importance of maintaining as optimistic an outlook as possible to try to buoy her spirits, even when she might have been tempted to give up and give in. Hope is a most precious commodity for the cancer patient, often very hard to find and, when found, dearly valued.

So much depends, of course, not only on the nature and seriousness of the cancer itself, the degree of medical care, and the treatment options available, but also on the personality and emotional attitude of the patient herself. Although Erie had struggled periodically with depression during her life, she also was gifted with an irrepressible sense of humor, a highly unusual sense of upfront candor in her dealings with everyone she met, and a profound love of life itself and of those she people for whom she cared. She was not, to put it mildly, a shrinking violet or a shy wallflower. From the moment we first met in September 1975, at a law school keg party – "Hi. I'm Erie. Like the Lake" -- to her last breath in March 2017, she was like no one else I ever knew. One trait that we shared, which I know sustained us throughout our lives, was a sense of humor and an ability to laugh at ourselves, as well as the vagaries of life.

That sense of humor was a key ingredient in enabling us to live with cancer for 25 years together and enjoy life in the process. The primary source of our joy and hope for the future, of course, was our joint commitment to do everything we could for our boys. Nate and Dave were just 10 and 6 when Erie was first stricken. Erie was determined to do all she could to stay alive and recover so that the boys would grow up knowing their mother and enabling her to impart to them her values of caring for others and pursuing their passions. A major source of our support was the wonderful community of Mantua and Pine Ridge in Fairfax, Virginia, ten miles west of Washington, D.C. Mantua Elementary School was the heart of the community. We moved to Fairfax from Arlington, Virginia, in 1988 so that our young lads could attend the school. Erie and I, like so many of the neighborhood parents, were regularly involved in all school-related activities, including PTA, fund-raisers, sports, and a wide range of extracurriculars. The support we received from the teachers, administrators, and coaches during the elementary school years gave us real hope that we both could see our boys grow and mature as young adults.

I mentioned the roller coaster analogy to life with cancer, with ups and downs, slow climbs and rapid descents. It was more than analogy; thrill rides became a big part of our lives. As a family, we always enjoyed many different sports and outdoor activities. Erie decided, just five months after her initial diagnosis, that, since the cancer hadn't killed her, why did she need to worry about plunging downhill at 60 miles per hour on a heart-thumping roller coaster ride? So we began a new tradition of spending Mother's Day by going to the Busch Gardens to spend the day riding the coasters. Erie embraced the thrill with abandon. She truly was able to put her mind over matter and set aside her fears. In later years, as the boys became teenagers, we often went to ride the biggest, fastest, scariest roller coasters in the world, including those at Cedar Point in Sandusky, Ohio, on the way to Shockey family reunions, as well as theme parks in Toronto and southern California. The more Erie rode, the more she loved it. Pure exhilaration.

As her cancer receded into remission during the 1990s and we proceeded into the new millennium with our move to Sacramento, California, we were able to embrace life with a new appreciation for each day and adventure. One source of pleasure was Erie's love of photography. Our vacations were marked by Erie's passion to document every experience and scene. She had a gifted eye and skill for capturing the beauty of nature, both large and small, as well as the people who filled our lives, resulting in an amazing collection of photo albums that we enjoyed ever since. Being able to photograph each vacation, each birthday party, each gathering of friends, each family gathering for Thanksgiving, Passover, Bar and Bat Mitzvahs ceremonies all give her enormous pleasure.

In the late 1990s, as her initial illness faded, Erie continued to stay in touch with her Bosom Buddies support group. For several years, she signed up to participate with many of them in the annual Race for the Cure, a running but mostly walking event held on The Mall in downtown Washington, D.C. One memorable year, on an especially beautiful Sunday afternoon in the Spring, we joined thousands of breast cancer patients and survivors and their friends and families, including Vice President Al Gore and his wife Tipper. Many in the crowd, including our family of four, were clad in pink shirts to demonstrate solidarity in battling to find a cure for breast cancer that has touched the lives of millions of women and their families around the country and the world. Seeing so many survivors stand and walk together gives rise to the eternal hope that a cure, one day, will be found.

For many people, including many cancer victims, hope is often manifest in religion, which may play a critical role in providing faith that they will survive the illness. If that hope ultimately should prove elusive, at least religion can provide great comfort in knowing that God or a supreme power in their lives will care for them and their survivors in death. Erie and I were different. While she was raised in an observant, Conservative Jewish home and well-steeped in the religious beliefs and cultural traditions of Judaism, she always had a rebellious streak that began in her teenage years that led her to question conventional wisdom and beliefs. I, in contrast, had been brought up with no religious affiliation or practice whatsoever. I jokingly referred to myself as a member of the AAU-Atheists, Agnostics, and Unitarians. When we met as law students at Georgetown in 1975, Erie's Jewish identity was something new and completely different for me. As the relationship ripened into love and a decision to marry, we had to confront the challenge of how we would deal with the role of religion and Jewish culture, which was so important for Erie's family. After much deliberation and no small degree of angst, we decided to get married and told her parents that I would convert to Judaism. To our great joy and relief, they accepted our decision and embraced us, easing the path for my conversion. For the next 40 years, we enjoyed a great deal of love and support from Erie's parents and the rest of her family. We sent the boys to Hebrew School, each one celebrated a profoundly moving Bar Mitzvah ceremony at the Western Wall in Jerusalem, and both Nate and Dave later on had Jewish observances at their weddings. Thus, Jewish traditions and culture have been an important part of all our lives.

And yet...when it came to the subject of death and end-of-life decisions, neither Erie nor I had a traditional Jewish belief in God, the eternity of the soul, or an afterlife. Part of the reason why our marriage worked so well was that we shared common views on many things, including the overriding importance of life itself. In other words, the most important thing we shared was caring for and loving one another and our families, while trying to live ethical and respectful lives within our community. The focus was exclusively on helping one another during our lifetimes, with no thought or concern for what would happen after we died. I attribute much of this to the guidance set by my own mother's example. She was perhaps the kindest, most caring, and ethical human being I have known, yet religion played no role in her life whatsoever. She treated people kindly because she believed that was the right thing to do, as her own parents had taught her. When my mom died in 1980, soon after our marriage, her legacy and her spirit lived on, first through my sister and me and through Erie, who was fortunate to spend valuable time with her before she died, and then through our sons, even though they never were privileged to meet their wonderful grandmother. I like to think that her spirit endures through our two young grandchildren whom Erie, like my mom, sadly, never got to meet. For Erie and me, in our belief system, the absence of religion or an expectation of heaven or an afterlife simply was never a factor. We always understood that religion is essential for so many people, especially when dealing with a life-threatening disease, and we never questioned the validity of those beliefs for others. It simply was not a part of our lives.

The subject of hope took on a very different dimension following Erie's recurrence in 2012. While Erie and I were devastated in 1992 when she initially was diagnosed with metastatic breast cancer, she survived, and our lives in many ways prospered as we had a newfound appreciation for life itself over the next two decades. In time, as the boys grew, we came to regard her cancer as a thing of the past. All our hopes for one another and our boys were realized. Life was good. So, it came as a great shock in 2012 when we learned that the cancer had recurred, this time impacting her bones and threatening to attack her critical organs. After we consulted several leading oncology experts; we quickly had no choice but to accept their unanimous conclusion. Erie's condition was terminal. She would die, at some point, from the Stage Four metastatic breast cancer recurrence. All hope vanished, at least initially.

We engaged in many long discussions with one another and with our boys and the rest of our family. As her caregiver, I was crushed and didn't really know how to respond or what to say. Erie was just turning 60 and still had so much vibrance and zest for life that it seemed unfair to have this dreaded disease rob her of that opportunity. One prominent part of her personality, however, was that she was incredibly tough. She didn't want a great outpouring of sympathy. She didn't want to feel sorry for herself. She was prepared, once again, to endure the pain and trauma of radiation and chemotherapy treatments. Through our consultations with her medical oncology team, led by Dr. Helen Chew at UC Davis, Erie realized that the prognosis, while terminal, was not an immediate death sentence. And she was determined to fight. While hope was a precious commodity in limited supply, she still had many reasons to live.

I have always been most reluctant to tell others how to live their lives, so I offer the following thoughts by way of one example from which others might benefit and perhaps incorporate into their own approach to caregiving. Erie and I were completely open and honest with one another about her medical situation and how we expected it to impact our lives. And, once we had talked through our emotions, fears, and concerns, we decided to be equally candid with our sons, our family, our close friends, and our work colleagues. This openness, for us, was extremely liberating. Everyone knew that Erie had a limited time left, though no one could say how long. The support we received, in return, was immeasurable and gratifying. Aided by Dr. Chew's straightforward though empathetic advice, we realized that we did, in fact, have some time left with one another. As it turned out, Erie lived for more than four years after being told of her "death sentence" with the recurrence of cancer.

Knowing that our time together would be limited, we focused on the most important things first. Fortunately, both Nate and Dave had embarked upon their careers and were independent and self-supporting, which pleased us enormously. We decided, however, that we needed to get serious about those always nagging  end-of-life planning decisions. We retained the services of an attorney to draft and execute wills, trust documents, and advanced health care directives to make sure that whatever resources we had would be apportioned as we wished and that we could exercise control over end-of-time decisions. I had continued to work at the U.S. Department of Justice for the first five months after Erie's diagnosis, and that work remained very demanding of my time and attention. After several months, however, I would come home in the evening to find Erie exhausted from her treatments and alone for far too much of the day. This just didn't seem right or fair to her. As her caregiver, I just wasn't giving her enough care and support. We took a hard look at our financial situation and agreed that I should move up my retirement as quickly as possible so that I could spend more time with her. Happily, with great understanding from my colleagues at work, I was able to retire in August 2013 at age 62, rather than waiting until I turned 65, as I previously had planned. That decision was absolutely the right thing to do. For the next three years, I was able to provide most of the care that Erie needed, including frequent medical visits, taking care of everything around the house, and, most importantly, being able to spend time with Erie, who was most appreciative.

Erie provided one major source of hope and optimism for the future. She really wanted to fix up our house and backyard, even though realizing that she would not have all that long to enjoy it. In her loving and caring way, she wanted to leave our home as a comfortable legacy for me after she passed away. We tapped into retirement and other funds to undertake a major renovation of our backyard, and we also renovated our kitchen and bathrooms. Each of these projects gave Erie great joy to participate in the planning and to see the finished product.

There were two more important activities that provided Erie with hope, optimism, and a real purpose and passion to pursue. The first was to plan and go on several family vacations, with Erie's camera always in hand. As we had discovered, if mom and dad offer to cover all the expenses, the boys were willing to come along. The most memorable trip was our first cruise, up the Inside Passage from Vancouver, B.C., to Glacier Bay in Alaska. We never thought of ourselves as "cruise" people, as we always had planned our own vacations, but it was quite nice to have all our needs met while Erie could rest comfortably in our cabin. The scenery and onshore adventures were a blast. Erie was delighted, as were we all.

The second source of hope and joy was pure Erie. We had traveled to Yosemite National Park several times and fell in love with the incomparable scenery. Erie decided that, even though "cancer sucked," there must be a silver lining. Because she always wanted to enjoy the sights of Yosemite in a convertible, she decided that we should get one. And so, we did - a silver 2006 Toyota Solara convertible, which she promptly named the "Silver Lining." We bought a license plate holder to match. The day after I retired, the two of us headed out on the highway. We drove from Sacramento to Houston to visit Erie's parents, then on to New Orleans and back home. We decided to avoid all interstate highways and all fast-food restaurants. The trip took 27 days, with 6,200 miles of nothing but sunshine, blue skies, and Sirius XM radio blasting away. We visited many national parks and other sites of interest. It was a very special way to realize that we still had time to enjoy our lives together. To this day, I drive the Silver Lining at every opportunity, with the top down, relishing our time together.

# Hope And Heartbreak

## By
## Cindy Bowden

My hope was immediate and constant the first time Randall was diagnosed with cancer in 2016. It was there for Randall the moment I looked into his questioning eyes after Dr. Mackrizz said "the cancer." For years, I had relinquished more and more responsibility at home to my husband. He loved and cared for me and I rejoiced in it. I was able to focus on us, on my graphic design career, and later, on becoming an elementary teacher. We did anything and everything to make each other happy. With his first cancer diagnosis, I just took charge. My number one goal from that day on: to make sure we both kept positive attitudes and stayed hopeful. After being admitted to MD Anderson, whenever I talked with our moms or siblings or friends, there wasn't a doubt in my mind that Randall would beat this disease. My faith in God and in my husband was strong. We had a fabulous circle of family and friends who supported us through those eight months. My siblings, Brian, Amy, and Deidre, my niece Hailey, nephew Sebastian, my cousin Tammy, Aunt Nancy, and sister-in-law Patti were also a great source of strength and support. Randall's mom, my step daughters, our grandchildren, his brother and sister, aunt, and cousins would call and text to say hello or offer words of encouragement.

Hope was a little more elusive two years later in August of 2018 and throughout the next two and a half years. The 12-month follow-up PET scan, showing a tiny spot in Randall's pelvic bone was such a shock to me that hope was taking a backseat; to that and to anger. Randall's hope and faith in Dr. Isabella Glitza and her team to stop the metastatic melanoma was there from the start. The outline she wrote for us during our first visit contained several detailed treatments, the last of which were full body radiation and chemotherapy. I'll admit,

I had my doubts, with the "Metastatic melanoma has no cure and a 20% remission rate," periodically running through my brain. Hope was easy to have at the beginning of a treatment and harder to hang on to after the scans showed the treatment had stopped working.

Randall was first treated with immunotherapy in Houston. The immunotherapy worked! It stopped the cancer from spreading while he was undergoing the treatment. In between these treatments, blood was drawn both locally and at MD Anderson to determine whether or not Randall's body could handle the next treatment. Dr. Glitza stopped this regime after four treatments; which was the maximum number of treatments safely possible using immunotherapy. The hope was that Randall's own cells would start fighting the melanoma cancer.

Immediately after the immunotherapy treatment, targeted radiation was used for the original spot on the pelvic bone and two additional that were showing in the scans and one on his right humerus. Gamma knife procedures were also used shortly after Randall's diagnosis to eliminate and/or halt small, specific spots of cancer from growing further.

Next up were the three separate clinical trials each in which he was enrolled for a minimum of 12 weeks. During these clinical trials, we traveled to Houston weekly for the treatment itself or the blood work necessary in between treatments. The clinical trials consisted of medicines not yet approved by the FDA. Randall would joke that he was MD Anderson's guinea pig. Each time, the clinical trial would initially stop the cancer from growing. Eventually, the cancer would start to spread again and Dr. Glitza would try to find the next clinical trial for which Randall would qualify. In fact, the cancer grew more aggressive during the third trail and Randall was exited after only 10 weeks.

COVID-19 shut down the Clinical Trial department at MD Anderson from March 2020 through the end of the year. Weekly blood work appointments and scans continued with Dr. Oches in Granbury and showed the cancer was progressing. Dr. Glitza made the difficult decision to try a fifth immunotherapy treatment on Randall during this time because his body responded so well to this type of therapy. There is a reason that no more than four treatments were given to patients. This rule was put into place because a patient's body could not handle typically handle a fifth dose, and Randall's was no exception. His bloodwork showed extremely high kidney numbers, fighting the effects of the immunotherapy and Dr. Glitza and Dr. Oches worked collaboratively and combated this kidney level fluctuation with steroids.

Randall started with taking 5mg of Prednisone each day, gradually worked his way up to 40mg a day, and then down again. When he was back down to lower steroid dosages, his kidney numbers shot back up and the months-long process started all over again. After the second regiment of Prednisone, Randall's kidney numbers stayed at normal levels.

Prednisone is a wicked steroid to live with. For months, Randall's disposition was not the same, his face and body were bloated, and he was easily fatigued. We were both working from home and I made calls to my mom while Randall was resting or working during these months, because for the first time in our marriage, Randall was not acting "like himself." It was a scary and frustrating time for me, compounded by the fact that Texas and other parts of the U.S. were being shut down because of the unknown that was COVID.

When travel and medical restrictions lifted, Randall qualified for and was enrolled in a fourth clinical trial. Much like the first three trials, the drug or combination of drugs seemed to work combating the cancer, but eventually the cancer would start growing again. Getting our hopes up and then finding out the treatment was not able to put the cancer into remission over and over was testing my faith and little by little, diminishing my hope. It was harder and harder to get excited about new trials because Randall was "probed, poked, and prodded" weekly, and sometimes daily—his words, not mine. He did not voice his frustrations until this fourth trial, but I could see the misery in his eyes during all of the clinical trials. It's a feeling of helplessness that I cannot possibly explain, watching the pain he went through during this cancer battle and not being able to ease his suffering. All I could do was stand by him, stay positive, and support the plan Dr. Glitza implemented.

Dr. Glitza at MD Anderson ran out of clinical trials. Randall's cancer was spreading and for the first time, we started seeing tumors. Knowing Randall had cancer and actually seeing the cancer were drastically different for us both. For all intents and purposes, Randall looked healthy on the outside. The tumors were painful in more than one way: a painful physical reminder in that he was able to lay on his back or side and sit down for only short periods of time. The tumors were also a painful visual reminder that the cancer was in nearly every part of his body. For almost 5 years, while combating two forms of stage 4 cancers, Randall had no outward, physical signs. I think the lack of tumors affected our outlooks. We were so sure he would beat this! He looked good, he wasn't in pain (because of the cancer), and he was able to work full time.

At our last appointment with Dr. Glitza, she scheduled two weeks in mid-March of full-body radiation treatments targeting several areas. There was still hope! The radiation could put the cancer in remission. After the first 5 days, the tumors started shrinking and after the second week of radiation treatment, they all but disappeared. Randall was thinner, but not experiencing the awful pain he had prior to the treatments. I found myself wondering why we waited years to try this and, at the same time, kept hearing the mantra, "Our last treatments will be full body radiation and chemotherapy," in my head.

Turns out, this radiation would be the last treatment MD Anderson had to offer Randall. Dr. Glitza wanted these two weeks of radiation immediately followed up by three chemotherapy treatments at home in Granbury. This was going to work! The morning of March 22, 2021, Dr. Oches gave Randall his first of the three chemotherapy treatments. It went well at her office and he returned home to work virtually. I was still working full-time as a paraprofessional, leaving the house each morning before Randall woke and coming home that week to him resting. He looked thinner by Thursday and when I left for school, he asked if I would make an appointment for that afternoon because he was having trouble breathing. It must be his oxygen levels because of the chemotherapy. He looks good, but is just exhausted and has lost some weight because of this back-to-back treatment and travel.

On Thursday, March 25, Dr. Oches said she was recommending hospice care. She told us she was stopping the chemotherapy treatment. In that moment, you could've knocked us both over with a feather. The treatments worked. Randall was relatively pain-free, he was able to sleep, the visible tumors that were treated with radiation were gone. I asked why she couldn't wait and see what happened after the next scheduled chemotherapy treatment in four days. She replied with emotion that she thought Randall would not survive another treatment and that his body just couldn't take any more. Randall had brought his FERPA paperwork to the appointment for her to sign. For the first time since the fall of 2016, he was taking time off work to rest and recuperate in hopes to beat the cancer. He died at home in the early hours of April, 7, 2021.

# Using Hope

## By
## Diane Linick

Thinking back, I understand now how embracing hope began after my husband's cancer diagnosis and how it fluctuated throughout his cancer journey. In 1997 my husband David had a small lesion on his right upper back removed. We learned that it was considered invasive melanoma with superficial spreading. Quarterly body checks were to be scheduled. In 2002 at a routine body check David's doctor took a small tissue sample from his left upper back. It was a second invasive melanoma. The quarterly body checks were to continue. During those years several other samples came back clear.

In 2008 David was bothered by itching on his back. Being the health-conscious person that he was, he set up an appointment to see his dermatologist. David's doctor did not like the color or shape of a mole on the left side of his back and took a small tissue sample from the area. Two days later David's doctor called to tell us that there were melanoma cells found in his sample. Due to the appearance and David's earlier superficial melanomas, David's dermatologist informed him that he needed a dermatologist surgeon to make a much larger incision for an additional biopsy of the area. He was equally concerned about leaving wide margins.

The following week at The Cleveland Clinic (The Clinic) David had the extremely wide and deep incision to locate and remove other questionable cells to help with  staging the melanoma. We were advised at that time to begin looking for oncologists associated with hospitals or clinics which had specialists in melanoma treatments on staff and were involved in melanoma studies and trials, in Ohio and out-of-state. The strategy was to have the oncologists examine David and study his records. We set up appointments and had consultations with hematologist oncologists in Cleveland, Columbus, and Pittsburgh. Our family in Ohio, as well as out-of-state, searched online for other contacts who would look at David's test results and respond to us if a consultation with them was recommended. Based on our family's notes and our own notes we decided to work with the oncologist at The Clinic.

At David's first appointment at The Clinic, we received much melanoma information and were provided with possible approaches to monitor David's condition. This provided David and I hope because David was starting the new phase of his cancer battle with options. David was told to return to his dermatologist for quarterly check-ups. These regular appointments involved several small tissue samples which all came back clear. The test results gave us hope that the surgery had likely removed or contained the malignancy, even though it had concerning dimensions.

At one of David's future exams, the dermatologist felt tenderness and a small bump in one of his armpits and David was in his oncologist's office that week. The Clinic oncologist followed up on David's case and ordered a PET scan and other diagnostic scans, procedures, and tests. He explained to David that often malignant cells travel to the lymph nodes. There were several lymph nodes that caused the oncologist concern. The medical team feared this would be proof of metastatic malignant melanoma in the lymph nodes. The test results came back prompting the need for a surgeon to perform a biopsy and the removal of all the lymph nodes from that armpit. David and I remained hopeful that both interventions, the large incision on his back and then the removal of the remaining lymph nodes in that same armpit could slow down the progression of metastatic melanoma. However, following the earlier excision on his back, I remember the doctor telling me in the waiting area that the growth was wider and deeper than expected and that a very large incision had to be done to provide David protection from the melanoma spreading. I was also worried that the cancer would possibly find its way into the blood stream from the lymph node.

This is when David first said out loud that he was losing hope that his cancer wouldn't metastasize to more places and organs in his body. We had a long talk with our lead oncologist at The Clinic. He spoke clearly as he gave us an overview of present malignant melanoma treatments. David requested printed information about all tests, drugs, and ways that he would be receiving his various medications and the purpose of each, and of course possible side effects. The oncologist explained that there is no true cure. At that time, they were using interferon- alfa. It is a substance made in a lab, a type of cytokine and type of immunology that provides additional help with an individual's natural interferon. In cancer interferon often helps keep cancer cells from growing and may possibly help kill cancer cells. Interferon is made naturally by our white blood cells, and everyone has them.

The Interferon therapy began in the fall of 2008, with high doses 4-5 times a week for about 4 weeks. This depended on how David's body would handle the "jump start" dosage given through an IV drip. Even after having been fully informed of the side effects and possible treatment setbacks, David was eager to get started! We reminded ourselves that interferon was the best immunotherapy for melanoma at that time. Extreme fatigue and fevers that brought on chills and night sweats began immediately after starting the therapy. Dosage was re-examined regularly and changed when needed. Occasionally, the doses were sometimes canceled. David was upset and less hopeful as this beginning process was taking longer than he expected. Step 2 in his interferon therapy was more manageable and was used in the ensuing months. David was taught to give himself interferon injections daily at home. He was fortunate that the project he was currently working on for his client allowed him to work from home instead of commuting to the NYC office. David was appreciative of the company's flexibility and understanding. He was on the phone, sending emails, and faxing papers nonstop. This helped fill his need and hope to live as normally as possible. Other than management David was able to keep his privacy with clients. I offered to give the injections to David but was glad to hear him say that he preferred to do it himself. I knew that it was a way for him to feel in control of a part of his treatment.

At each oncology appointment the doctor would start out discussing that week's blood work and gently, but honestly remind us that with Stage IV Melanoma there was no cure at the time. The purpose was to extend his life. David assured the doctor that running had taught him to constantly challenge his body! He would now see how far he could go in this cancer battle. We loved being parents and adored our new status as grandparents. Thinking of his children and grandchildren gave David all the motivation and hope he needed. When David would get upset when medications and trials had to be modified, I would show him pictures and videos of our grandchildren, a gentle reminder of the goal of his battle. I tried to give us both a chance to reminisce about all the great memories of watching our children grow. David and I had a long-standing tradition, starting back at college. Every few years the two of us went out to dinner with the sole purpose of making fun predictions of what each of us would be doing in the next few years. These evenings started out with a recap of the last few years. We would be amazed at what each member of our family had accomplished, often far more interesting and exciting than our guesses. I hoped that the photos and predictions would let us share in our pride of the family we had become. The last thing David wanted to hear from me were a bunch of promises or false hope after facing a setback in his treatment schedule.

In the summer of 2009, the oncologist discussed a trial that was being run at The Clinic. If David was accepted and if he agreed to it the doctor would apply for a spot for him. No promises were given, and we understood, but it provided us a glimmer of hope. This trial was done at home. There were very detailed directions with complicated pill scheduling. Naturally, given the warnings of possible results and side effects, life was becoming more uncertain. Even with a positive attitude it was tough keeping up the fragile hope we had. When the trial was over and hadn't made a difference, David was disappointed, yet continued to ask for more options.

There were no new trials available to him until September 2009. There were lengthy discussions about possible cardiac risks when receiving this therapy, Interleukin-2 (IL-2). First, he would be meeting the oncologist who was running a new trial at University Hospital in Cleveland. At this time, while waiting for the new trial to begin, David admitted that he was truly worried that nothing had been helping him and he had doubts that this extremely dangerous trial would succeed. Unfortunately, the University Hospital trial that took place in the ICU wreaked havoc on his body and had to be stopped earlier than had been planned. I could now understand why he wanted no one to have false hopes in the beginning. He didn't want to let us all down.

# Hope Fights Fear

## By
## Sonja McCaughey

Hope came slowly. Hope came when I made it to the hospital chapel where it was quiet and away from other parents who were afraid just like I was. Hope came when I finished praying.

The medications were doing their job for Nikita and killing the Acute Lymphocytic Leukemia. Hope came when Nikita was heard laughing at something silly as little girls often do. Hope came with every smile and every cute hat she wore and with knowing that she would soon be celebrating her 10th birthday. Hope came with a lot of prayers to stop the fear of her not getting to grow into a young woman. Hope came from every conversation with other parents who were on the same hospital floor and who talked about their fears in their children's fights against cancer. The nurses brought hope each day with their calm demeanor and knowledge of how to handle children when they were in fear, in pain, or just not feeling well that day. The best hope was hearing the doctors explain that your granddaughter will be able to have children one day.

Hearing them say that lifted the dark cloud of fear and opened the opportunities for Nikita to grow up, have a career, and have the ability to have children of her own one day. The highest level of hope came from the knowledge that the entire medical staff was trained to adequately teach a 9-year-old about her cancer and how her care was going to be handled, step by step. They brought pictures and medical equipment that she could touch as they explained what certain equipment would do and why things had to be done in certain ways to battle cancer. The medical team wanted to make sure that Nikita understood her cancer and her treatment and, most importantly, that it was going to be a long time before she could go home. They encouraged her with information on the importance of eating the right food and how certain medications might make her feel. She listened with such intensity that I believe she understood she was going to be okay. They empowered her with the hope to live.

Nikita was not quite 11 years of age when she was released from Walter Reed Medical Center and the family finalized their plans to move to Florida. After her move to Florida, it was discovered that her port was not functioning properly, and she would need a replacement port. We were told that ports could stay in the body for up to ten years and now we have one that malfunctioned in a relatively short time. (Deep breath.) My daughter-in-law, my granddaughter, and I went to Saint Joseph's Children's Hospital in Saint Petersburg, Florida for the outpatient surgery (yes outpatient surgery); a one-hour procedure that insured the proper care for cancer treatment. Nikita did very well with the procedure and was wheelchaired out eating a bag of potato chips. Seeing her eating that bag of potato chips after surgery made me smile and hope continued to grow.

Hope diminished a bit when Nikita experienced headaches. There were times when she was exhausted and needed to rest. Her little brother grew impatient with her when she did not want to play like they used to. There were times when she would become very frustrated because she could not figure out how to put together a Lego toy. She became angry with her homework because it used to be easy for her, now it took her longer to figure out the assignment. We all learned very quickly how to redirect her and not get upset with her because chemotherapy was killing her cancer.

Every day of seeing her grow, smile, and start to play increased our hope for Nikita. Every once in a while, though, the tiredness would come across her face, sometimes fear. There were times when she was scared to play because she did not want to bump her port. She understood the importance of what the port meant to her life. Eventually, Nikita made the decision to play on a basketball team. Nikita wore a chest protector that protected her port if she was bumped into on the court.

She got bumped a lot and her hope grew stronger when she realized she could get bumped while playing basketball and she would be okay. She became stronger in her ability to survive cancer, and she became a fierce competitor again. Nikita is now 15 years old. She has been in a soccer league for several years and is in the school band. She lost her taste for basketball but who knows what sport she'll do next. We hear hope when we hear of Nikita's plans to become a doctor and that she wants to treat cancer patients. As long as she has the ability to look into the future, everything that she does increases our hope of her dreams coming true.

Nikita is aware that I am writing for awareness about her cancer and my experience as a caregiver to her family. I did not have any intentions of talking to her and giving her input. Nevertheless, once I made this decision it brought clarity to children that go through this experience. I asked her a few questions and some of her answers made me think about how profound her answers were. I asked her "what's the most important thing that you learned about yourself going through cancer and the treatments?" As I waited for her answer, I was imagining all kinds of answers but the response she gave made me appreciate her more and I saw more hope for her life within her answer; "I don't care what other people think about you." She believes cancer has made her a stronger person both mentally and physically. As many people stared at her for wearing a mask – pre-Covid, asking her questions about wearing a chest protector when she played basketball, and why she could not do certain things that most kids her age were doing she learned a more valuable lesson. Life will get better soon.

Nikita is still young, and it is too soon for her to decide where she wants to attend college, but while she was waiting for cancer to go into remission, she had made plans to be a doctor when she was nine. With her insight into people and the experience of having cancer, she will bring a different level to being a doctor. I asked her the question, "What is the best advice you would give to another child when they learn they have cancer?" She replied, "That it is going to get better soon, and the future will get better."

I struggled with my last question to her. I asked a tough question about her cancer, and I stumbled in asking her for fear that I may introduce a thought or a fear to her. I was not sure I wanted to hear her answer. "Are you ever concerned, or afraid cancer might come back? Her answer was strong! Her answer was confident! Her answer brought me more hope than the doctors, the prayers that I said every night, and it reduced my fear and gave me more hope. Her answer was "no." Sometimes the power of healing is within the person who is healing.

I was a police officer for many years. Most times, officers would take the initial report, and if an additional investigation needed to be made the report was sent to the detective division. When I made detective to the Major Crime Unit investigating crimes on children, there would be officers that would want a follow-up call on the case they initiated. At first, I became annoyed that an officer would call. However, I quickly learned that if the case was impactful to them, they needed to know the conclusion to the case they started. There were many cases that I would follow up with an officer to inform them how well they did, or how the case concluded. Not only was this an opportunity to maybe teach an officer, but most importantly, the conclusion gave them the closure of how well they did which allowed the investigation to conclude with a positive ending. Police officers want to know how a case ended. It gives all of us hope that what we are doing is right. In one particular case, I was working with a crime scene technician who was photographing several children that had been abused. It took a few hours to photograph the injuries. There was some discontent from this person about why so many photographs had to be taken. One injury may need several photographs to show the injury. I explained that when the injuries heal the evidence may be gone and the children may forget what had happened to them. Eighteen months later the case went to trial; however, the perpetrator took a plea agreement to 15 years in prison for aggravated child abuse for the injuries that they inflicted to their own children. When I left court, I called the crime scene technician to tell them the photographs solidified the case. The children did not have to testify, and this person would be released from prison when the youngest child would be 18 years of age. Hope comes in all directions. When we trust the system, the experts who are wanting a good ending, and the faith that our work is good, we all heal with hope that we are doing the right job when called upon.

# Support and Lessons Learned

## By
## Elizabeth Hapner

Supporting your child through cancer treatment is a unique voyage. Each child has a different perspective on how to travel this road. Kyle was very private about his illness, rarely posting anything on social media or discussing it with anyone outside his treatment team and immediate family. Rarely did I even see him cry after the initial shock of his diagnosis. I just knew if he wanted to go in his room and be alone or simply go see his Kylie, he was struggling. As well as I knew my son, it was still a learning process as he proved to be much stronger than I had ever imagined.

Many people choose to use CarePages or CareBridges to keep a running journal of their cancer journey and to keep friends and extended family apprised of the current situation. Kyle did not want to do that, choosing instead to control the dialogue through social media posts when he felt the desire to inform friends. Most of his posts related to his faith or simply to activities in which he had engaged. Little was actually said by him about his treatment.

After Kyle's diagnosis, we first saw a nutritionist at Moffitt. All we were really told was that he should consume as many calories as possible. Our understanding had been that sugar should be avoided and that he needed protein. Apparently, that is not the case. Boost was recommended and Publix stocked their pharmacy at Moffitt with it at a reduced price for patients. Unfortunately, Kyle did not like it in the cardboard containers in which they carried it so we had to get it at full price at other places.

Next on the agenda was the supportive care physician, in an effort to manage Kyle's pain and minimize the effect of the disease on him. His oncologist quickly reached the point that he felt medication management for pain would better be handled by the supportive care physician. His supportive care physician was wonderful. Suggested were acupuncture, counseling, massage therapy, and medication. Because of his fear of needles, Kyle was not willing to try acupuncture. He tried massage therapy once but did not feel it was sufficiently helpful to warrant traveling across town for it. Counseling was attempted several times, but he felt that discussing the situation just made it worst.

Throughout his illness, Kyle was resistant to discussing his feelings about it. Honoring his wishes, I did not press him to do so. His supportive care physician tried several times but was unsuccessful in changing his mind, after the initial few visits he tried. We both felt that Kyle would benefit from the practical advice he would likely gain through the young adult support group but he was not willing. Although I would have liked to revisit our lifetime of memories, in his mind, that would have entailed acknowledging that his life with us would shortly be coming to an end. Hospice provided him with a bear with a recorder inside to create an audio memory for me, but he never recorded anything for me on me. Instead, we just concentrated on spending time together and creating additional memories.

Even though I wished he had handled that aspect differently, it was not my choice to make. I feel certain that he did not think about what he would or would not be leaving behind for me. Being supportive and upbeat was the key for Kyle so that is the tact I always took. His girlfriend at the time was very emotional about his illness and it irritated him to no end that she imposed that emotional burden upon him. His father was having great difficulty dealing with the reality of his illness and was hampered by that fact.

The best support for Kyle, aside from Kylie, his treatment team, and me, came from friends who simply included him in activities, making accommodations for his physical restrictions without ever making an issue of them. This treatment made him feel "normal" for a short period of time. His best times during his illness included going to Florida State football games with his close friend, Jeff, and others and going to the local Hard Rock casino to play poker. I was willing to fund pretty much anything that brought him enjoyment. Friends of mine also provided Kyle with opportunities for experiences that brought him joy during his illness. Use of a box for Lightning hockey games and club seats for Tampa Bay Buccaneer games, with sideline passes were among the gifts bestowed on him.

Colorectal cancer is a very painful form of cancer. It greatly impacted Kyle's ability to participate in activities he had previously enjoyed. At times, the simple act of visiting with a friend or family member was too much for him. I had visions of taking a number of trips with Kyle during the balance of his shortened lifetime but that proved to be unrealistic. While we did take various trips, I had to make major adjustments to my expectations of the activities in which we would be able to engage.

My mother was Kyle's only living grandparent by the time of his diagnosis and she was well into her battle with Alzheimer's. While she outlived Kyle by nearly two years, I never told her of his illness or death. My sister and Kyle's cousins were spread out across the United States, but they also kept in touch. Kyle's half-sister, nieces and nephews, and two step siblings, all on his father's side, visited occasionally and communicated with him fairly regularly, With no real family locally, I quickly learned to accept all offers of help from my friends.

Because cancer is generally a prolonged illness with extensive treatment requirements, it is often difficult for others to constantly be available for support. While I was able to provide the ongoing, consistent support, I did not hesitate to call on friends for support during crisis periods, not only for Kyle's needs but for myself as well. Simply knowing that others cared and were available to us was a tremendous source of comfort for Kyle and for me. Do not hesitate to call on your friends and family for whatever you need in this journey. Just remember that it is far easier for them if you assign them specific "tasks." Many who mean well simply do not know what to do or say but are happy to assist when asked to do something in particular. Do not forget to take care of your own needs. You cannot provide for your child if you are ill or emotionally overwrought. To be available to support Kyle, I had to make certain I remained healthy and so I was careful to keep my medical appointments for basic needs, such as prescription refills. Getting adequate rest was also essential because it assists with the emotional fatigue as well as the physical. I did not choose to participate in a support group, either during Kyle's illness or after his death. With Kyle's death occurring during the early part of the pandemic, only remote support would have been available. I chose to simply rely on my faith and the support of my friends.

Kyle attended the last Bucs game of 2019 and the last Lightning game of 2020 before the pandemic shut down all sports. Club seats and sideline pregame with the Tampa Bay Rays were made available to me to take him and a friend of his. Friends also arranged for Kyle to get a video message from Jameis Winston, then the Bucs quarterback and a favorite of Kyle's from his playing days as quarterback for Florida State. He also received numerous autographed footballs, photographs, baseballs, caps and other memorabilia from local athletes, including the Tampa Bay Rays. And he greatly enjoyed his time spent at my friend's beach condominium even though he was not up to fishing or actually going down to the beach.

The other source of support for Kyle was his deep and abiding faith. Although he did not get to church often after his diagnosis, he prayed several times a day and we discussed the fact that we ultimately would be reunited again. Kyle knew that I would have traded places with him in an instance to give him more time on Earth. The Hospice chaplain also came by several times prior to the pandemic closures. While Kyle was happy to have him pray with him, he still did not want to talk about his situation in great detail.

Many longtime friends of Kyle's kept up with him through text, Instagram, Facebook and phone calls. This was really the only form of communication during the last six weeks of his illness because of the pandemic restrictions. Kyle hated going through the last weeks of life without the ability to see his friends or even watch live sports on television. The silver lining was that the courts were closed so I was able to spend all my time with him, without court interfering. Fatigue had really set in by then as Kyle's body began to shut down but during his waking  hours, we watched a lot of movies and talked. His pain caused him to be awake more at night and less during the day. Not going to court permitted me to alter my sleep patterns to more closely coincide with his.

# Chapter 4:

# Saying Goodbye

# Saying Goodbye
# Rituals and Normalcy


## By
## Linda W. Devine


Friends tease me that I am the person that goes to the most funerals. That may be true, and in reflecting on the notion of saying goodbye, I thought about this gentle poke. My internal rule (I have too many of those, but at times they help me flip the proverbial coin) is that I make every effort to attend an engagement that will not or cannot be replicated. And funerals are such events. I learned this from my father, who quietly did not miss a beat when he heard someone had passed. He and Mom might send food from their country butcher shop to the family home, and then he would be off to the viewing or the funeral service.

Familial goodbyes for me have been powerful in visceral ways, just as they are with many people. Losing family members, whether biological or chosen, through death alters one's framework of the world. My first profound goodbye was to my Dad. He passed at 66 years of age, far too young and poignantly just after he handed the reins of the family business to my brother Michael. I was in my late thirties and pregnant with Danny, child three. Dad had been on a progression of life support measures for nearly six weeks, and I vacillated on when to fly to my childhood home, given his precarious condition. Mom and I had a frank discussion about when to make a trip, and she said she would let me know when it was time.

And she did. I arrived at Lorain Community Hospital on the south shores of Lake Erie on a late dark fall night, and I checked in at the reception desk. Lorain is my birth city as well as Dad's, and on more than one such visit, including that night, the reception volunteer remembered me. Those connections and feelings of normalcy are comforting at any time, but all the more significant in times of apprehension and uncertainty. I went to Dad's room, and there with my sister-in-law Nancy, who was also pregnant, we stood on opposite sides of his bed. He was intubated, yet he looked at me with that "I know you are here" look, his green eyes seemingly satisfied. Then he lifted both arms and patted our respective tummies, saying hello and goodbye to the boys he would not get to meet in person. We let him gently fall asleep and then went to the family home. He did not awake again, and we often wondered if he stayed with us long enough to say goodbye to all his children.

Twenty-eight years later it was Mom's time. I watched her in those last weeks, tossing fitfully in the middle of the night, talking to whom I think was her Mom and Dad, and to my Dad. There was some issue, likely forever unknown, that finally she reconciled, and the fitfulness subsided, and her demeanor relaxed. In the mornings when she was awake, she would tell me that she had vivid dreams and about the people who were on her mind. I would like to think she had met her biological father, something she had told me she wanted throughout the six years she lived with me. The sweetest hello into the hereafter I think I witnessed was her talking to a small girl. She asked me if I could see her, this small girl. I hope that it was my older sibling that she lost just days after giving her birth in 1952. Baby Girl Wryst, as she is forever known, had a medical issue that in today's scientific advancements could have been remedied, but at that time it was not to be. How lovely it was if these three are now celebrating, catching up on eternity.

The passing of my parents and how my family said their goodbyes was entangled and strangely comforted by a combination of ritual and the need for normalcy. Catholic roots run deep in my family of origin, and even though I am not a card-carrying member, my cradle Catholicity created a path for saying goodbye to my parents. There is a Catholic prayer asking for a peaceful death, and I had not thought much about it until my walk with Mom in those final few weeks.

My brothers visited shortly before her passing, and she rallied, like so many do, to spend time with her boys. She was fully present during the Blessing of the Sick that the priest from Saint Paul's administered, and after he left our home, she joked with my hubby Dave that she'd likely give up sex for Lent, a normal jousting that occurred during the Lenten season between the Protestants and Catholics in the family. The night before my brothers left, she sat in our living room, eating bits of barbeque chicken and pizza, watching the bantering, and Face Timing with cousins, spouses, and grandchildren with a serene gaze. I often wonder what she was thinking, or if she was already moving on in some regard, knowing that the family she created seemed to be faring well. The following morning, she insisted on dressing and pushed herself to use the regular toilet, an act that Tavia, her aide, and I made possible knowing it was her dignity getting the best of her. She then ate a regular-sized breakfast, sitting between her boys, creating normalcy for them, just as she had for 60-plus years as their mother. It was then time for sleep, which was now taking up 20 to 22 hours each day. She said goodbye to her boys in her regular way, and then we tucked her in.

Tavia was an important part of maintaining normalcy. She had been a constant in Mom's life, and although Mom could be tough with her, Tavia persevered. Professional caregivers like Tavia taught me a lot about maintaining normalcy and finding ritual in the every day. During those last weeks when we bathed Mom in bed, refreshing the clothes and linens, we joked with her that this activity was part of her "Spa June" (her name) experience, and that we were there for her spa treatments. We got Mom giggling and making wisecracks, as was usual for her. Those are sweet memories for me.

Over that next week her sleep was peaceful, and by Wednesday she was no longer awake. A peaceful passing was something for which she always prayed, and physically she morphed into what I can only describe as beatific - simply beautiful, with luminescent skin that seemed to lose its imperfections. The Hospice practitioner had counseled me on what I may expect in terms of her appearance, which would degrade as dialysis had been discontinued. She was surprised, too, when she saw her, marveling at her smooth, pink skin and lack of edema. With one long out breath, she simply slipped away from us on Saturday afternoon.

Rituals guided us over the next weeks as we planned her funeral Mass, choosing scriptural passages with personal meaning, and selecting the clothes in which she would be buried. My brothers and I were fortunate: over our lifetimes she had slowly divested herself of possessions and made her wishes known. The normalcy she created with the closure of this life dovetailed with the rituals she held dear, helping me to say goodbye and to weather difficult hours.

I think it may be a Polish Catholic thing, or perhaps just an old time custom of many groups that was passed along in my family, that we keep every Mass, holy, remembrance, funeral, viewing, or other named card that one picks up when they call on the deceased and family. I have yet to go through Mom's box, and my box has now been taped shut and the second has been started. The cards are of every variety, loaded with traditions. I do not know at this writing whether I will keep them, but for right now, they are tucked alongside family Bibles and other mementos of transitions. I suppose they are reminders of those who have walked before me to wherever one walks next. And, they are symbolic of the farewell. I thought about those cards in a recent visit to the Museum of Natural History in Washington, D.C. There is an interactive exhibit about a group of early humans and the cave in which they lived. By examining the dirt and bones, scientists have determined that this group took care of their sick person, well into his elderly years. And when he passed, they layered his grave with colorful flowers and carefully positioned his body in a pose of comfort. Like my memory cards, the dirt and bones tell stories of how we say our goodbyes, lovingly help our people with their transitions, grieving their loss for this life, and hoping for unification in what lies beyond.

While we pass along as solo travelers to the next realm, we live presently in a world filled with people. Good people who pop up at the most important and sometimes unexpected times. We may be saying goodbye to those we love, or we may be grieving for a way of life we once knew. My Dave is alive and faring very well at the time of this writing, and I hope there are many more memories that we can make together before we part this life. It is the friends and strangers who made the goodbyes to my past and my people bearable. It was the Moffitt Cancer Center clinical trial coordinator who caught me in a corner of a hallway, crying with abandon as Dave was getting measured for radiation treatments. And the Moffitt cashier who let me slip into the cafeteria for coffee after hours and then did not charge me for it, as she knew I was there late after Dave's brain surgery. It was co-workers who kept projects and meetings, big and small, going, taking my place and filling in, as the cancer schedule was not of my own making. It was my prayer group at First Reformed Church of Tampa and the prayer groups of my friends that let me know others were thinking about us, lifting us up in their petitions. It was the traveling nurse who told me "it was time" to call Hospice, holding back the tears so she could be brave for me. It was Dr. Noh, Mom's primary care physician, who sat with me for an hour one Friday evening as I decisioned my way to Hospice care. It was the Hospice nurse who sat with me in our garage and told me in the most kindly straightforward way what would happen when dialysis was discontinued, leaning into her own experience with her Mom. And it was the two men from Segel Funeral Home, who let me linger with Mom before they gently covered her with cloth and zippered the carrying bag, quietly and skillfully moving her on a stretcher down our driveway to their vehicle.

There have been so many good people. And I am sure there will be many more. And I hope that I am one of those people to others, helping them navigate the rituals, creating the normalcy, and being the person who helps link the present with the future in measured, kind, and thoughtful ways.

# Speaking Goodbye

## By
## Charles Shockey

The first time I had to say goodbye to a loved one was to my mom, who died in February 1980  after a seventeen-month battle with metastatic colon cancer that had spread to her liver. Because the liver was impacted, we knew from the time of the diagnosis in July 1978 that her condition was terminal, so my sister Kate, my wife Erie, and I all had sufficient time to prepare for her death and to make sure that the time we spent with her was precious and meaningful. As a newlywed and recent convert to Judaism who had started attending services at our synagogue in Alexandria, Virginia, I was exposed for the first time to a somewhat structured and religiously based process of confronting death. In many ways, the prayers and words of the service were foreign to me, yet, rather surprisingly, I found great emotional comfort in listening to and reciting one prayer, known in Hebrew as Oseh Shalom. The prayer, always sung, has a haunting and beautiful melody, and the words and music moved me to tears as I thought of my mom. Loosely translated, the prayer asks "May the One who brings peace in the high places also bring peace to all mankind. Amen." This is a wonderful sentiment, regardless of one's religious beliefs. The traditional Jewish prayer said at the time of death and at subsequent memorials afterward is known as the mourner's Kaddish, a prayer derived from the ancient Aramaic language. Curiously, the Kaddish does not mention death or dying, but instead extols the greatness of God. Saying Kaddish has been a very different experience for me, considering my non-religious upbringing, but I find comfort in reciting the words of the prayer. For me, it was a way to say goodbye, while looking to the future and committing to living our lives to the memory of those we have lost.

Twelve years later, I again faced the prospect and fear of saying goodbye, this time to my wife. Erie was only 39 when she was diagnosed with metastatic breast cancer, but we immediately had to confront the distinct possibility that she might die. With two young boys to raise, this was a most unsettling development that shook both Erie and me to the core. While we tried to maintain a positive outlook on life, we had to prepare ourselves emotionally for the worst-case scenario. I wondered if I might have to say Kaddish again, this time for the love of my life. Happily, Erie survived, as the cancer went into remission following extensive treatment and first-rate medical care, accompanied by the outpouring of love and support from family and friends.

Twenty years passed during which we were able to raise our boys and enjoy life in so many respects. Erie's cancer returned in December 2012, however, this time as a terminal illness. So, we embarked, once again, on the difficult process of preparing to say goodbye. Thanks to the magnificent care that Erie received, we were blessed with four years together before the end arrived. This gave us time to reflect and decide on what steps we wanted to take to redirect the course of our lives in whatever time remained. This reexamination involved financial decisions to prepare for the future, as well as pragmatic changes such as projects to renovate our house and yard.

The most significant and traumatic reassessment was the emotional challenge that the recurrence of cancer presented. We talked at great length about what Erie's death might mean, how it might play out, and what kinds of medical treatment she would, and would not, tolerate. We also talked about what my life would be like without her. This was particularly painful for me, as I preferred to repress all thoughts of carrying on alone after she had departed. But Erie, always the pragmatic realist, insisted that we talk about that scenario, as it was no longer an abstract question, but a certainty. These were difficult and emotionally draining times for us and our boys. Every night as I drifted off to sleep, I wondered and worried about what horrible and saddening thoughts must occupy her heart and soul. What is it like to know that you are going to die? I wondered, too, what my life would be like, living alone after spending every day and night for 40 years with the woman I loved above all else in the world.

Because a terminal cancer diagnosis imposes so many difficult and often impossible demands on the patient, and because cancer takes over so much of one's life, Erie expressed an urgent need to try to exert an influence over those matters in her life that she could control, at least to some degree. Cancer sucks, she often said, but she was determined to fight it with every bit of strength she could muster. Cancer sucks, so, in fairness, there should be a silver lining. She found hers in buying our silver convertible, which we used to travel around California and the West. Cancer sucks, but at least she could get a prescription for medical marijuana, which she employed quite liberally. Marijuana, she found, did not remove the pain caused by the cancer, but it was the best way to minimize the nausea resulting from chemotherapy, radiation, and other cancer treatments. Plus, she had always liked getting high. So why not indulge, especially at this point in her life? Dr. Chew, her oncologist at UC Davis, could not write Erie the marijuana prescription, but she empathetically supported Erie in this and other decisions, recognizing the importance that Erie attached to having some control of her life as a cancer patient.

Erie also formed an exceptionally strong relationship with Dr. Nathan Fairman, a psychiatrist at UC Davis, who recently had joined the medical team at the cancer center. Erie had counseled with psychiatrists throughout her adult life to treat depression. Although Dr. Fairman's primary role was to prescribe medications, Erie found that he had a genuine willingness to listen and guide her through the mental and emotional trauma of facing cancer. Despite his initial reluctance, she convinced him, through the force of her personality, to meet with her regularly to talk through her concerns, in addition to writing prescriptions for her meds. Dr. Fairman also invited me into the conversation on several sessions, which was beneficial to all of us. In fact, Dr. Fairman later invited us both to address his graduate school students at the UC Davis Medical School to provide them with a cancer patient and caregiver perspective on facing critical end-of-life decisions.

Erie also learned that Dr. Fairman was working actively with the California State Legislature to consider a death-with-dignity law, based closely on Oregon's law. If enacted, this would enable terminal cancer patients in California to obtain a prescription for end-of-life medicine allowing the patient to exercise the choice of when and how to die, rather than letting the pain continue unabated until death occurred. For Erie, this was critically important. She wanted to know that, if her condition deteriorated to the point where it was excruciating pain and discomfort, she would have the means to control her own right-to-die. Erie worked with Dr. Fairman and many others to persuade the State Legislature to enact the "End of Life Option Act," which took effect when signed into law by Governor Jerry Brown on January 1, 2016, with the support of more than 75 percent of Californians. When the time came to say goodbye, Erie would have a say in how the end would transpire.

During the three years of her active oncology treatment from 2013-2016, Erie and I took advantage of the opportunity to spend as much time as possible with our sons and their girlfriends, who would soon become their fiancées and wives. Nate and Felicia would visit from New York when they could, and we saw Dave and Mandi in Sacramento regularly. We also made a point of seeing as many close friends as possible, both from California and from our many years in Washington, D.C., and the East Coast. As I had discovered many years earlier with my mom, each visit was precious, as no one knew whether that would be the final goodbye. We continued to travel to New York for our annual Thanksgiving visit with Erie's family and to Houston for Passover each Spring, as her aging parents had become too frail and infirm to travel. The visits with her parents, by then in their late 80s and early 90s, were quite difficult emotionally for us. They realized that they would outlive their own daughter, who was nearing the end of life in her early 60s. This wasn't fair, as we all knew, but cancer and other terminal diseases have no sense of fairness. We had no choice but to carry on with life. And so we did.

In late 2015, Nate and Dave each became engaged to the special women in their lives, Felicia and Mandi. This brought great joy to all of us, especially Erie. Yet, as with so many aspects of life with cancer, the engagements also brought along a sense of sadness, as Erie knew that she would not live long enough to enjoy seeing the lads progress into marriage. Like my mother, Erie knew that she would never have the exquisite joy of becoming a grandmother. This brought a profound sadness, as she surely would have "kvelled" in the joy of having grandchildren. In her inimitable and life-affirming style, she told the boys that, while she did not expect to live long enough to attend their weddings, she was determined to throw a dual engagement party for them at our Sacramento home. The party, in December 2015, was a glorious celebration of our sons, their fiancées, and Erie. It was her way of saying an early goodbye to our immediate family and dearest friends.

As her cancer spread and progressed throughout her body into 2016, Dr. Chew continued to prescribe new treatments, but the side effects of chemotherapy grew more difficult and painful, and the efficacy of each new chemical cocktail lasted only for a few months at a time. Dr. Chew mentioned on one visit that UC Davis had a pain management program that might be able to offer some relief. Erie and I met with the head of the program, Dr. David Copenhaver, who described a surgical operation that would insert a "pain pump" near her spine to dispense micro-doses of narcotics on a regular basis, which Erie could control. Because the pain levels in her lower back and spine had become so extreme, she agreed to the procedure. This was, if not quite a lifesaver, a miraculous device that greatly reduced Erie's chronic pain and enabled her to rest much more comfortably for the final year of her life. Having Drs. Chew, Fairman, and Copenhaver work together to address Erie's cancer and do everything possible to alleviate the pain was, in a word I rarely use, a godsend. While the cancer marched inexorably onward, Erie had a great team helping her cope.

By the summer of 2016, other symptoms arose, including one cardiac episode that required us to call the Emergency Medical Team and have Erie transported to UC Davis Hospital in downtown Sacramento. The Emergency Room doctors admitted

Erie to the hospital overnight to monitor her heart condition. Her heart stabilized the next day, our 38th wedding anniversary, and Erie firmly rejected the doctors' advice to stay in the hospital. She insisted on being released because she said it was the cancer that would kill her, not her heart. Her best friend from law school was visiting, and we had planned a retreat to one of our favorite places, the Mendocino California coast. Erie would not be denied. We made the trip. The scenery was spectacular. The Mendocino Botanical Gardens were stunning. And we returned home to a very big decision. Erie decided that she was through with chemotherapy and active treatment to attack the cancer. She wanted to end oncology treatment and transfer into Hospice Care. She informed Dr. Chew of her decision, and the doctor promptly made the referral. I fully supported Erie's decision. Thus began a new and final chapter of our lives together.

I knew very little about hospice before then. I had the vague notion that one typically went to a hospice facility somewhere. And I assumed that, once referred, the patient frequently died within a very short time. Those notions, as I soon discovered, were largely outdated. Like many large hospitals and other medical centers, UC Davis has its own hospice program, run by a medical administrator and an extensive, well-trained staff that specialized in end-of-life treatment. To qualify for a referral to hospice, the treating physician must certify that, without continuing active medical care, the patient was likely to die within six months. Erie's hospice care was entirely home-based, which is what Erie most wanted -- to die at home, not in a hospital or care facility.

The very first day of hospice care, a team came to our house and provided a comfortable bed in our downstairs living room that would become Erie's resting place for the remaining seven months of her life. With the referral to hospice, the responsibility for Erie's medical care transferred from Dr. Chew and the UC Davis cancer center to the UC Davis hospice team. They were incredibly wonderful in every respect. I quickly learned that a principal benefit of hospice is not only to make the patient as comfortable as possible, but also to provide relief to the caregiver. I had been feeling great anxiety as to how well I could care for Erie full-time at home, including giving the right medications, cleaning all tubes and equipment, and taking care of her daily needs such as bathing and dressing. My anxiety instantly evaporated. Hospice took care of her every need. Staff would stop by several times a week at least, including visits from nurses and home health care assistants. I was freed up to spend more pleasant and meaningful time with Erie in conversation, watching television, and relaxing, without feeling that I was alone responsible for her medical needs. Hospice, truly, was a blessing.

Erie still had a strong will to fight on as long as possible. Nate and Felicia were to be married in August 2016 in upstate New York. To our great joy, we discovered that we could travel there for a week to attend the wedding. The UC Davis hospice team arranged with a local hospice organization in Dutchess County, New York, which set up a bed and provided all the necessary equipment for Erie to receive the treatment she needed. Her ability to be with Nate for his wedding exceeded our greatest expectations. The entire weekend was a very special time for us, with Erie's family, many of my relatives, and our close friends all gathered in celebration. After the wedding, we traveled back to Sacramento via Houston so that Erie could see her parents one last time. This visit, as expected, was very touching and tearful, as they prepared to say goodbye to one another after more than 63 years.

Upon our return to Sacramento, the pace of life began to slow considerably. Erie's mobility diminished, along with her energy level. Thanks to Dr. Copenhaver's pain pump, she was not in great pain or discomfort. We spent most days resting and relaxing at home and occasionally seeing visitors, while the hospice team and I took care of her daily needs. Erie continued to communicate with Dr. Fairman, the UC Davis psychiatrist, and requested that he prescribe for her the end-of-life medications authorized by the new California law. While she did not know that she would use the medicine, she felt very strongly that she wanted to have it available in case her condition worsened to the point that the pain and nausea became intolerable. After several meetings and consultations as required by the law, Dr.

Fairman wrote the prescription and, along with the pharmacist, went through the detailed steps and procedures that would be required. While I could prepare the medication, Erie must be capable of administering it herself. Because we wanted to have this new law succeed, we were extremely conscientious in making sure we knew exactly what to do, if that time ever arrived. As it turned out, it never did. The hospice nurses were able to control her pain through other means, and Erie was greatly comforted by knowing that she had the legal power to take control of her life and die with dignity on her own terms. Later, after her death, I carefully packaged up the unused medications and returned them to the custody of UC Davis.

The start of 2017 was an extremely emotional time. Not only were we prepared to say goodbye to Erie, but we also were busy preparing for Dave and Mandi's wedding, set for March 11, 2017, in downtown Sacramento. Because we had no way to know how much longer Erie might survive, we had extensive discussions about the wedding plans. Happily, everyone was unanimous that the wedding should go ahead on schedule, no matter what. This is consistent with Erie's view, which I share, that life must go on for the living and that death is a natural part of the "circle of life." Even as Erie's strength was sapped and she drifted into longer periods of rest and sleep, we were determined for the wedding to proceed. We understand that many people do not share this view and believe that any celebration much be postponed for a period of mourning after a death. This was the traditional custom and practice in Judaism, as well. I certainly pass no value judgment. I only know that Erie and I, along with our sons, were completely open in discussing our feelings about this most sensitive topic with one another. Fortunately, none of us had any reservations about the decision to proceed with the wedding.

As it turned out, the timing proved to be a blessing. Our families and friends gathered in Sacramento for the wedding weekend, and everyone close to Erie had the opportunity to come to the house and spend a little personal time with her. Although she was confined to her hospice bed in our living room, everyone was able to share their final thoughts or simply to hold her hand and kiss her goodbye.

Because her health had declined rapidly in the days before the wedding, we agreed that she should rest at home, rather than attempt to attend the ceremony itself. While her absence was evident, the ceremony was beautifully and sensitively conducted by our dear friend Steve Lewis, who led Dave and Mandi through their vows. Despite not having Erie there in person, her love and spirit were felt by everyone present. The wedding was a beautiful, touching affair that brought great joy to all.

Four days later, on March 15, 2017, the Ides of March, Erie passed away, quietly and peacefully in her bed at home, as she had wished. The hospice nurse controlled her pain until the very end. Dave and Mandi stopped by that afternoon to say their final goodbye, as they headed off on their honeymoon. I reassured them that mom would have wanted them to go ahead with their honeymoon, despite the surreal nature of having a wedding and a funeral in such rapid succession. They had done everything possible to care for her in a loving manner as her life ended, and the focus should now be the start of their lives together, always guided by Erie's spirit and memory. Nate and Felicia were with me that evening, as Erie breathed her last breath. They, too, were able to have a meaningful and emotional goodbye. We all held hands and touched Erie for the last time as she slipped away.

In early April, Erie's family gathered in the Houston area for our annual Passover holiday. Her parents were there, as well, and we said Kaddish and spent an afternoon recalling the role that Erie had played in each of our lives. Erie and I each had made the decision that, upon death, we wished to be cremated, rather than buried. This was a controversial decision, especially within the Jewish faith, but the decision was ours alone, as I explained to her family. They understood our view and accepted the decision. On April 22, 2017, Earth Day, we held a memorial service and celebration of life for Erie at the Women's Empowerment Program in downtown Sacramento. She had worked there for more than a decade, helping women and their children fight the challenges of homelessness, abuse, and addiction. Among the many heartfelt tributes, the most moving were from several women who said that they would not be alive if Erie had not intervened in their lives and helped them to overcome their challenges. This was their chance to say thank you and goodbye to Erie. Two of my nieces ended the ceremony with a beautiful guitar playing and singing rendition of "Somewhere Over the Rainbow / What a Wonderful World," performed initially by the Hawaiian artist Israel Kamakawiwo'ole. There were no dry eyes. It was the perfect way to say goodbye.

# Celebrating Randall

## By
## Cindy Bowden

The first time Randall had cancer, in 2016, neither of us talked about saying good bye. He did insist on updating our living wills, powers of attorney, and other written wishes, but it was as far as we would go in that direction. During his fourth week-long chemotherapy treatment, in February of 2017, Randall shared that he wasn't sure if he could "take anymore." I sat by his side day and night, willing him to live as I had during the first three weeks of this treatment regimen. Failure was not an option—he was one tough hombre (OTH). Later, Randall would tell family and friends, "One night, as I was lying in the hospital dying, looking at my wife, I wondered, 'if my wife and my friends think I am the toughest person they have ever met (OTH); and I give up, what hope does that give them when they face adversity?" He made it through.

At the end of his second battle, after fighting stage 4 metastatic melanoma for 19 months, on March 27, 2021, Hospice came to the house for our "intake" process. Randall wanted very little support from the organization; he just wanted me in the house. Hospice protocol is that a nurse visits at least once a week. We saw a nurse twice during those 11 days. Randall's stamina was waning and it took two or three days for him to explain our bill situation, how to access online bank accounts, and how to take care of the yard. After one of these tutorials, Randall stopped, looked at me and said, "Cindy, you are the best wife, EVER. I mean it. You are the best wife, EVER! I don't know how I got so lucky; marrying you." I remember thinking his eyes looked so big and sincere in his thin face. Much like my mother, all I ever wanted to be was a good wife. Somehow, he knew just the right thing to say that day.

Like so many others across the nation, the pandemic prevented Randall's family from visiting during the two years before he passed. In March of 2020, Dr. Glitza, Randall's metastatic melanoma oncologist at MD Anderson, wanted Randall to stay isolated and he worked remotely for Tarleton State University for the rest of the year. Randall's mom, Barbara, his sister Cindy Anne, and his brother Les scheduled a couple of trips to Texas in 2020 but weren't able to fly down; either because of Dr. Glitza's directives to have Randall in isolation or because of COVID travel restrictions. By the time he was in hospice care, people were able to travel and I asked Randall if he wanted anyone to fly down. He was adamantly against seeing people because he didn't want family and friends to remember him ravaged by cancer. He said, "I'd rather they remember me healthy and active; how I looked at the Louisville Ironman over a year ago."

Randall was able to sleep quite a bit and didn't eat much over the next week. The days went by quickly and were simply surreal. Here was this man who accomplished every mental and physical task he set out to do; yet his body was unable to stop the cancer. I used to marvel over the fact that he could figure out any problem that would come his way. On Monday, April 5, he looked at the hospice nurse and said, "I don't want to do this anymore." Then he looked over at me and I saw the exhaustion in his eyes. He had battled stage 4 metastatic melanoma for 2 ½ years and was tired. He died in my arms at 2:25am on April 7, 2021.

Randall's wishes were to be cremated and his ashes to be spread at the Three Rivers Confluence in his native state of Idaho. I turned to Randall's sister Cindy Ann, and while I was in a daze for the months following his death, my sister-in-law took over and coordinated his Celebration of Life. Cindy Ann lives in California and did everything to make Randall's celebration a success. She found B&B's and hotels in the small towns of Kooskia and Kamiah. Cindy Ann worked tirelessly selecting the date, sharing travel and accommodation information, and planning the actual celebration. Randall's family made the trip from other parts of Idaho, California, and Florida in July 2021 and my relatives flew in from Texas, Colorado, and Florida.

Our friendship means more to me than Cindy Ann will ever know. She supported me in those horrific months after Randall's death, taking that weight of planning Randall's celebration off my shoulders. She took on this responsibility having lost her older brother, while I struggled to go to work and keep up with my own basic needs.

Randall's Celebration of Life was on Saturday, July 10, 2021. Thirty family members and close friends made the drive to the confluence on a beautiful, sunny Saturday. While walking down to the river and along the bank, Cindy Ann encouraged us to pick up a river rock. We wrote our farewells on the rocks and tossed them into the river. My brother-in-law, Kelley, said a prayer and I scattered Randall's ashes in his fly-fishing spot. Cindy Ann proposed a toast to her big brother Randall, all of us with Jack and ginger ale (his favorite cocktail) in hand. His uncles sang and played guitar and we released butterflies. One butterfly remained on my shoe and another on the ground by my feet for a minute or two before taking off. I took that as a sign that Randall was with us and appreciated our celebration. Over the years, I would say, "Everyone loves Randall." and judging by the outpouring of support we received during both of the cancer "wars" and the support I've received throughout the last year; I've never been more positive of it. I appreciate all of our family and friends for keeping Randall alive in our minds and hearts by sharing his jokes, telling his stories, and marveling at his accomplishments.

# A Journey's Closure

## By
## Diane Linick

As I reflect, I realize that saying goodbye may come in different ways along the journey. Pay attention to your loved one's clues, even if you are not ready yourself. I believe you must respect the patient's wishes about personal issues. "Life is Good" was our motto throughout our marriage, even before the brand began. Whenever David or I were down, the other used this saying to keep us hopeful. This was ultimately a part of David's "goodbye" to me during his final weeks, as well. David knew that I would understand that he had reflected on his life as well as mine. He was now focusing on the good life he lived and encouraging our family to continue to live by our motto. Yes, there were always going to be difficult life challenges, but we should appreciate every day as they happen. That is what he had learned and wanted for us. I continue to wear my many "Life is Good" (LIG) t-shirts and feel especially calm when I wear one of David's "LIG" hats. It feels like we're walking together, having easy conversations. I remember David's positive outlook about all that life had given us and I smile.

When a Stage III melanoma becomes a Stage IV metastatic malignant melanoma it's hard to know what to think. When David started his journey with his oncologist in 2008, he was overwhelmed with medical facts and the talk of numerous scans, clinical trials, types of chemotherapy, and various new specialists who would be members of his Cleveland Clinic oncology care team. As he learned about possible treatment plans and their side effects, he felt lost in this new and scary vocabulary. After the high dose interferon therapy and self-injections of interferon were reduced or stopped early and David regained his strength, he began the process of planning his legal and business affairs, something David understood and could control. As an attorney, and faced with his reality and diagnosis, David knew that certain legal documents would be needed for the hospital and that personal family affairs would need to be put in order at some point of the journey. As upsetting as this was to me, it was what David personally needed to address at this time. Most pressing to him were household and family financial matters. David had always discussed these with me and explained his routines and showed me where important papers and lists were in his office. However, David enjoyed taking care of these responsibilities. Other than when he was traveling for business or had his shoulder surgery David never accepted my offers to help. In the final months, David knew it was time now to teach me his ways. It definitely was a worry for him until he supervised me for several months. I am forever grateful he had the foresight to prepare me and reached out to trusted family members who would later guide me through the financial and technical aspects of running my household.

As with my sister, I was not ready to acknowledge what I considered to be negative thinking, while there was still hope for possible upcoming clinical trials. I soon realized how important David still felt about his main role in our family. When David's final round of clinical trials began in the summer and fall of 2009, I needed to remember what I had learned from my sister's Hospice nurse. David needed for me to now begin the conversation to exchange our goodbyes. Providing opportunities for David and me to have peace of mind and closure would be beneficial to each of us going forward.

I had known that my sister Ellen and I needed to share our fears and sadness about losing each other. I also knew she was worried about her family and our parents, and I promised to be there for them always. Ellen understood, but at that time she was overwhelmed and needed reassurance. We continued our discussions over her last few weeks. I was afraid if we had this exchange too soon it would seem like I had no hope for her (similar with my thoughts about David). I knew she was doing everything possible to remind her family and friends of their beautiful memories shared over the years.

Sadly, my brother Alan, who was a cancer survivor, died alone in his house from cardiac arrest. No one was able to say goodbye. Fortunately, he had been at a wonderful family event with all of his children and grandchildren the night before. Personally, I'm grateful that just the week before his death we had one of our most memorable phone calls. We didn't talk regularly, but I am very glad we did then!

In the case of my parents, I feel that they were content when it was their turn to say goodbye. They were the ones who actually helped me during their own last days. They guided me through their example. They told me what I had meant to them and I, in turn, was able to express my feelings to each of them. As I've said, my father was at peace with his leaving us. He had told us daily how proud he was of our family. He just wanted to be surrounded by family when he said goodbye and we reassured him that he could count on us to take care of my mother.

During the calm before the two storms (chemotherapy trials) David was busy trying to complete his legal/business part in a major project for work. We were both quite anxious and worried about side effects before starting the latest trial that was going to be done at the nearby University Hospital. Being in the ICU was beyond our comprehension. He was afraid of being drained from the rigor of his treatment and unable to focus when at home before the start of the weekly treatments. Therefore, David was determined to finish projects at home and for work before the trials started. I thought that this would be an opportune time for David to see our friends and thank them in person for their support. David realized he could tell them how much he valued their friendship. I chose eight huge, beautiful chocolate/caramel apples. I was able to make times with our friends the following Sunday afternoon. They were each waiting in their driveways for us. We put our windows down and David could see the love in their faces. David was able to present the apple and say thank you and together they exchanged memories and goodbyes. One of David's closest friends and his wife met us in their driveway with pastries and drinks for a quick snack together. It was a beautiful day. Yes, David was exhausted but grateful he was able to enjoy his short but meaningful visits.

Over twelve years later and our friends, at random times, still tell me how special the visits had been and how much they needed the closure. Personally, I needed to be a participant in those interactions and the closure for David's journey as much as our friends.

# Saying Goodbye

## By
## Sonja McCaughey

How do you say goodbye to someone who has cancer and is only nine years old? I listened to what the doctors were saying statistically about ALL. Even after six years of that first diagnosis I still hear those doctors say statistically how this cancer can aggressively come back when she is older. Out of all of my grandbabies, Nikita is the most compassionate and has a gift of discernment. No one wants to say goodbye to such a beautiful person. God has a purpose for someone with her compassion for people, for life, and for those that are around her. It never occurred to me to think about saying goodbye to her. It never occurred to me to think about her not being here to grow old. It did make me think about her opportunities of becoming a mom herself, but the doctors assured us she will be able to. Will her cancer treatment stop her dreams from happening? Once she became acutely aware of her cancer, she decided that she wants to be a doctor when she grows up. Will the cancer treatments prevent her from her achieving those goals? Saying goodbye is not just about somebody's final days on earth. It's also saying goodbye to opportunities that may not occur because of what chemotherapy does to the body in the battle against cancer. But, how do you say goodbye to opportunities that have not happened? God blesses us with talents and maybe the talent we think we have is not the talent God wants us to use.

I will not say goodbye. I refuse. I have not had enough time with her. I need more time and more memories. I want more hugs and conversations about how her day went. I want to hear about her dreams and how she plans on making her dreams come true. If I prepare myself to say goodbye, then I have accepted the fact that I will not get to hear or see her plans come to fruition. Saying goodbye was not an option when I learned Nikita had cancer.

I did have to say goodbye to my grandson. When the family moved to Florida my little buddy was ready to live with his family. I had to say goodbye to my full-time Grammie parenting for him. The house was quiet again. I was cooking for one again. I would have to wait for visits to drink ice-cold blueberry tea and spaghetti with mounds of cheese on top. I will wait for him to come to my house where we can make lemon bars together. I will miss him counting each lemon bar to see if any are missing from the last count. I will miss Levi trying to find the right spot to catch a fish and will miss watching him struggle to get to the cypress stump where he sat looking at minnows. I watch his cartoons. I would be saying evening prayers alone, and now I was planning on going back to school to finish my degree.

Cancer makes a lot of things more difficult. Nikita is in remission, and she got to ring the bell as she left the hospital with a clean bill of health. She will be in the care of doctors for many years to come, but to ring the bell was like a survivor acknowledging the battle was won. I really wanted to be there when she rang the bell. It would have brought me closure to see her and to hear the bell being rung; I was there from the first day she went into the hospital. However, this was her journey and her saying goodbye to cancer.

Unfortunately, we did have to say goodbye to the family unit. My son's and daughter-in-law's marriage did not survive the strain of being apart during a debilitating situation. Differences in parenting became more difficult when dealing with the dynamics of how this family was separated by cancer. Who worked harder at getting Nikita healthy? We all did.

Saying goodbye to cancer is super easy. Saying goodbye to all the worry that cancer brought was easy. But saying goodbye to the family unit was hard. I understand the dissolution of the marriage, and I will leave it at that. I know God has a plan for all of us and maybe this was a test of what He has in front of us. Nikita and Levi are doing well and both parents have remarried. Aside from what cancer has done, everyone is happy.

# Life During Treatment

## By
## Elizabeth Hapner


Just before Kyle's diagnosis, I had made the decision to sell the large house in which he had been raised and move to a condominium. As a single, middle-aged woman, I was tired of the maintenance required for a home with an unscreened pool, large yard, and several oak trees, one of which was a Grand Oak more than one hundred years old, With the move, I went from a neighborhood fifteen to twenty minutes from the main campus of Moffitt to one on the other end of town. However, that move put be close to Tampa General Hospital which is where Kyle would go in the event of a medical emergency. Kyle's lease was up approximately a month after his diagnosis and initial hospitalization, so he moved in with me shortly after his release from the hospital. My condominium was also far closer to his work.

My initial plans to renovate the condominium went by the wayside with Kyle's diagnosis.  Faced with the uncertainty of out-of-pocket costs for Kyle, and the need for a peaceful environment in which he would live, renovations had to be postponed indefinitely. In the midst of his illness and treatment, the condominium elevator had to be replaced. Because of errors by the elevator company, the process took nine weeks instead of the expected three. Since my unit is on the top (fifth) floor, this was a definite hardship for Kyle who then had to climb stairs after treatments, A good friend from high school made things much easier by offering us the use of his beautiful waterfront condominium on the beach but when we returned, we learned that the elevator was going to be out of service again for two to three weeks several months later. Do not hesitate to accept the generosity of friends throughout this battle. Above all else, be adaptable, because you do not know what will occur.

Kyle did not experience nausea after treatment but could not tolerate cold items, even a cold bottle of water, for several days after a treatment. Extreme fatigue was a continuing issue. Neuropathy varied. As descendants of George Washington, Kyle wanted to visit Mount Vernon and Washington, DC so I planned a trip for April 2019. When we arrived, the weather had taken a sharp turn and was cold and rainy. Scheduled for a Segway tour the afternoon of our arrival, we were not prepared for the cold and Kyle's neuropathy made it very difficult for him to grasp the handles of the Segway in the cold. A guide came to his rescue with some heavy gloves but we were still cold and wet when we finished the tour. Future trips involved preparation for all kinds of inclement weather, which proved advantageous when we went to New Orleans in December 2019.

With a chronic or terminal illness comes logistical challenges of a different sort as well. First is insurance coverage, essential for treatment. Because Kyle was consulting with M.D. Anderson in Texas, as well as Moffitt, Medicaid would not cover his care there. Medicaid in Florida requires two years of disability before fully taking effect. In the interim, prepayment was required, with submission for reimbursement after approximately $850.00 in out-of-pocket exclusions per month at that time. Kyle's life span was limited to the point that his COBRA did not expire before his death nor did Medicaid fully kick in.

Social Security disability is also essential, if like most young patients, your child is not working. For minor children, the benefits will be based on the parents' earnings. For an adult child, it would be based on that child's earning record (if sufficient). For a serious diagnosis such as cancer, Social Security disability is generally granted on the first application and can be done without an attorney. You must gather all the medical records to document the diagnosis and severity. Despite his Stage 4 diagnosis, however, I was required to take Kyle to the Social Security office because they said they could not match his Social Security number to his driver's license and had to physically see him to match him to his driver's license photograph.

One of the best decisions I made was letting Kyle get a dog. Initially I had ordered a mini Golden Doodle puppy. The breeder made an error and thought we wanted a full-sized Golden Retriever puppy. Living in a condominium, that was not an acceptable option. Nor was waiting for another breed of puppies, given Kyle' life expectancy.

Off we went to Humane Society on Saturday afternoon. While I had in mind a small dog, twenty-five pounds or less, Kyle fell in love with a forty-five pound puppy. We traveled on to the local county shelter, where Kyle was not enthralled with any of the many dogs available. Insisting that we had to go back to the Humane Society for the dog he wanted, we arrived after adoption hours had ended for the day. The result was that we found ourselves back at the Humane Society thirty minutes before opening on Sunday morning to get his chosen dog, Kylie, as Kyle named her. Kyle dashed in the moment the doors open, fearful that the woman in front of us wanted "his dog."

Words are inadequate to express what a difference Kylie made in Kyle's quality of life. After any bad news was received, all Kyle wanted to do was go home to his Kylie. Never would Kyle go to his father's without Kylie accompanying him even when it added an hour to his travel time. For an only child, Kylie's love and unwavering devotion were priceless. When given paperwork by Moffitt to list his final wishes, his only one was that I keep his dog. Initially reluctant to do so, I honored his wish and Kylie, now seventy-five pounds, has been a great source of comfort.

Within a short time after we acquired Kylie, Kyle had a favorite blanket with a photo of her head on it that he always took with him to Moffitt, a silver charm in her image that he always wore and a pillow with her head on it. My favorite photo, which he wanted displayed at his memorial service, is one taken of the two of us with Kylie not long after we brought her home. It hangs proudly in my front hall. Whatever comforts you can provide your client through this process will be gifts you will never regret.

After approximately a year, chemotherapy quit working for Kyle. After more genetic and other testing, he commenced immunotherapy. A dramatic advance in treatment, immunotherapy has had life-changing results for some. There was only one form of immunotherapy available for Kyle. Unfortunately, he could not tolerate it. The side effects became progressively worse for Kyle and after several sessions, he went into seizures when immunotherapy was initiated. By November 2019, immunotherapy had to be discontinued. Testing showed that it was not really effective for him anyway.

The news that there were no treatment options left came the day before Thanksgiving, 2019. His wonderful oncologist was in tears as he imparted the news. The following week, his position had changed, and he determined that we would fight on. Medication was prescribed that we all hoped would prolong Kyle's time on earth. At that juncture, Kyle had accepted that his time on Earth was coming to a close, much sooner than any of us desired.

# Chapter 5:

# A Meaningful Life

# It's The Small Things

## By
## Linda Devine

My friend Al passed away this spring after living through the effects of Parkinson's disease. He was a brilliant academic, skilled in the deanly things one thinks about when "business dean" is conjured up in the mind, but his interests went far beyond the academy. Through the years, we had deep discussions about life, underscored, bolded, and in italics. That was Al. He always caused me to think about the essence of things. Why does this human behave in this manner? Why do we follow certain political leaders in this election cycle? And why does this pho taste so good?

Exploring the meaning of this existence is the ultimate "why" question. It is an ironic collision of circumstances as I think about living a meaningful life as I am leaving my full-time university employment in the coming weeks, mourning the loss of a friend, and considering what will be next. I sat recently in Saint Patrick's Cathedral, amidst the hauntingly beautiful Gothic architecture. I thought of my own First Reformed Church of Tampa which has little adornment. And then my mind flew to the elegant simplicity of Congregation Schaarai Zedek where my Rotary friend Jean was memorialized. And then on to the recent passing of Thich Nhat Hanh, a Buddhist monk who was known worldwide for his meditation teachings. And my thoughts turned to those I know who are not part of a faith community - some not religious at all - some who do not believe in existence after this life. Why are we here? What do we hope for in this relatively brief time on Earth?

Hubby Dave's cancer started my thinking on this topic in earnest. It was not my choice of timing, but sometimes the big questions present themselves at the most inopportune times. I was happily surveying my life just prior to his diagnosis, and wham. All changed in a moment. And once the initial shock and awe diminished, the questions started. Why Dave? Why me? Why does this have to happen now? What do we do? To whom do we need to connect? How do we rearrange schedules to manage treatment? What about work? How will the household budget hold up? What about the vacations we had planned? Will we have Christmas as usual? When can I visit Mom as she rehabs from pneumonia? Why do we have to go through this?

Why are we here? And so in 2014, I started my exploration about what would bring meaning to my life, now profoundly different. I am continually amazed by the diversity of human lives and the communities in which we reside, and the purposes to which we commit while we are alive and the legacies that may be left once, we depart. The people in my professional world have purposes around human growth and development of all types - intellectual, emotional, spiritual, physical - and in the best sense, a blending of these facets. We walk alongside students as they struggle and soar, offering appropriate coaching and tools and an occasional Kleenex. We sometimes think about salary and benefits, but that seems to be an episodic occurrence. I have friends for whom the accumulation of wealth is very important, and I observe as they tell the tales of deals gone well and bad, the ups and the downs, the fat times and the lean times. I have many friends who enjoy service encounters in industries of all kinds - real estate, banking, retail, and wholesale markets. They like the interactions and the satisfaction of processes gone very right and happy campers as consumers. Then there are family and friends who seem to work in shift schedule but sometimes are called upon to work inordinate hours with no clear end time: in an operating or emergency room, seeing patients, transporting the ill, fighting fires, in law enforcement. I watch people who create things: arts, crafts, wine, jewelry, stage sets, furniture, photographs, meals, flower beds, vegetable gardens, dog haircuts, nails that sparkle, clothing. The world is full of people who do countless tasks.

And some of those tasks culminate in big results. My friend Al led colleges of professors in three universities. The big idea of a St. Patrick's Cathedral was built by a person who imagined a spiritual respite in the heart of the island of Manhattan at a time when not much existed structurally besides woodlands above 50th Street. And St. Patrick? Parts of his life are largely unchronicled, but his impact has been felt around the world. I love the modern conveniences that big results make possible - effective medicine, safe food, transportation that can take me around the world, and technology which creates communication spaces so appreciated during Pandemic when we were relegated to home. These big results allow me to explore meaning in many ways. But as I watched the changes in Al and my Mom as they took the last turn in their journeys here, and as I created care for Dave and Mom, I realized that the truly meaningful came in the small things. One of Al's interests was drawing and painting, with an eye for the lines. I am not an artist, but I saw the enormity of thought in the very simple strokes of his art implements on paper. At first the finished products look, well, unfinished. But sitting with them, I saw how Al used the lines in sparse ways to create. He allowed the patron to explore the spaces between the lines and immerse in the why's of the figures.

Dave and Mom's care was bounded by the everyday: good food, medicines passed at appointed times, sitting, and watching the glories of the hours. There might be a car ride to fetch an ice cream on a nice day, or just to feel the wind. Bird watching became a source of conversation, particularly as the grumpy sand hill cranes made their nightly stroll past our home. Watching bad golf, too, was a favorite of Mom's, who never golfed but knew what poor golf looked like as the balls hit our trees, patio, and sometimes the house. She would also report the numbers of jets she saw pass in the distance, a barometer of the world re-emerging from COVID.

And, as our bodies begin changing in preparation for what lies ahead, our worlds seemed to get smaller. With Dave and Mom, relationships became larger as the stuff of this world receded in importance. The conversations became about times of long ago, the picnics and parties and gatherings, the visits with family and friends, the funny moments, the people to which we already bid farewell, the foods and meals of an earlier time, the hopes and prayers we have for the next generation of family. William Channing Ellery was a Unitarian minister nearly 250 years ago, and his words are among those that sustain me when I think about living a meaningful life:

> To live content with small means.
>
> To seek elegance rather than luxury,
>
> and refinement rather than fashion.
>
> To be worthy not respectable,
>
> and wealthy not rich.
>
> To study hard, think quietly, talk gently,
>
> act frankly, to listen to stars, birds, babes,
>
> and sages with open heart, to bear all cheerfully,
>
> do all bravely, await occasions, hurry never.
>
> In a word, to let the spiritual,
>
> unbidden and unconscious,
>
> grow up through the common.

This is to be my symphony. Little did I know at the time of Mom's changes that the seemingly small moments and actions would become the big things, the meaning makers, for me. And as Dave continues to enjoy good health, I relish finding meaning through happy, kind, peaceful moments with whomever I encounter. At the end of a project, a day, a life, I cannot think what would matter more: to create my life's symphony with the instruments of every encounter, no matter how small or seemingly insignificant. Because there is no insignificance, I think, in the human condition. We are all part of a greater plan.

# A Meaningful Life

## By
## Charles Shockey

"Depend on it, sir, when a man knows he is to be hanged in a fortnight, it concentrates his mind wonderfully." The English writer Samuel Johnson wrote those words referring to the impact of an impending death by hanging, but, in my opinion, his observation applies with equal force to a diagnosis of cancer. When we first learned that Erie had breast cancer in December 1992, our world came crashing down upon us. We were completely unprepared for what came next. We had very little idea of how we would make it through that day or the next, much less through the weeks, months, and years to come. Unlike some cancer patients and caregivers, we were fortunate to secure a stay of that execution, which eventually lasted for 25 years. In the instant aftermath, however, we found that we had no choice but to concentrate our minds, perhaps not wonderfully, but out of necessity. Erie survived for so long through her incredible fortitude and determination to live, combined with the unwavering support and love from our family and friends and the magnificent care she received from her medical teams in Northern Virginia and the Sacramento area.

Still, upon first hearing that she had cancer and that it had spread to her lymphatic system, we were lost in so many ways. I suspect that this feeling of helplessness is commonplace among those whose lives are stricken with cancer. After the initial shock, we immediately began to regroup. There were many daily living tasks that required our attention, especially looking after our ten-year-old and six-year-old sons. With help from her family, we were able to maintain some semblance of their normal school and play routines, which we felt was essential for their well-being. Once the immediate fear of death subsided, as Erie's oncology treatments kicked in, we entered a new phase of our lives together, no longer fearing death at any time, but instead learning to live with cancer as an omnipresent factor in our lives. We had no idea, of course, how long we might have together as a family, but we talked at great length about what mattered most to us. I would encourage others facing similar situations to take advantage of the opportunity to reevaluate their lives…to concentrate their minds and hearts, in other words, on what is most important, while putting off lower priorities to the side, for the time being.

I was fortunate to have a very fulfilling career as a trial attorney for the U.S. Department of Justice, working on federal court cases around the country on environmental and natural resource issues, especially those involving endangered and threatened species and marine mammal protection. I loved my job and my career. But I loved my wife and my family far more. I suddenly faced the prospect of having to curtail my career in order to care for Erie. We both knew that our rather idyllic suburban family life could end in short order. Erie also loved her work as a social worker in Fairfax, Virginia, helping emotionally and physically challenged and disabled high school students. As we both worked for public sector government agencies, we were blessed with supportive and understanding co-workers and supervisors who gave us the time we needed to rearrange our work schedules and assignments. Then we focused on how to set our priorities for the future, with a new understanding and appreciation of the precious gift of every day that we could share together. I believe that many others can do so, too, and gain some semblance of control over lives impacted by cancer

When Erie's cancer recurred 20 years later in December 2012 as Stage 4 cancer that had spread to her bones, we knew that our long stay of execution would end. Once again, we had to decide how best to make our lives together as meaningful and fulfilling as possible. This time, the outlook was markedly different than in 1992. Our boys had grown into fine young men, with promising professional careers and loving partners, so the principal concern of parenting vulnerable and innocent young children, which badly frightened us earlier, now had been alleviated. Still, Erie was not quite 60 when the terminal cancer card was played against her, far too young and vibrant to have to face death at a relatively early age.

She had become accustomed, as a cancer survivor, to expecting many more years enjoying life with me and the boys, even becoming a grandmother at some point. That dream now vanished. We had some important decisions to make. How did we want to spend our time? What would make our limited time together as meaningful as possible?

Much depended on her physical strength, as the cancer slowly spread throughout her body. Her primary medical adviser through this process was Dr. Helen Chew, an exceptional oncologist at the UC Davis Cancer Center in Sacramento. Through our dozens of trips downtown to see her and receive hormonal and chemotherapy treatments over the next three years, Erie realized that she still had time and opportunities to pursue the things that mattered most to her. She had retired from her job as a social worker for women experiencing homelessness and frequently the victims of substance and physical abuse in Sacramento. Yet she continued to stay connected with many of these women and their children through the Women's Empowerment Program. Erie's generous spirit, if anything, grew stronger as she was determined to offer as much care as she could, despite her own declining health. Just as Dr. Chew gave Erie hope that she could live a meaningful and productive life even as a terminal cancer patient, so, too, Erie wanted to share that feeling of hope with women who had to confront daily challenges of finding a place to sleep, protecting their children, and finding food and shelter. That incredible ability to focus her concerns outwardly is perhaps the single trait that earned Erie such amazing loyalty and love from all who knew her. That positive attitude provides a good model for others by focusing outwardly on others, as well as inwardly on oneself.

We also wanted to enjoy ourselves with family and friends. This included a  decision to break into our piggy bank of retirement savings and spend it now. Erie's father always pressed his children and grandchildren to live frugally and responsibly, keeping savings set aside for a "rainy day." Erie had to convince her dad that, with the recurrence of cancer and her terminal condition, the skies opened, and it was raining damned hard in our lives. Why not use the money we had available to fix up the house, to travel with our boys and close friends, and to enjoy a few more nice meals than we were accustomed to eating? And why not buy a used convertible, Erie's Silver Lining, to travel around California and the West with the top down, the radio on, and the wind in our hair, even if she no longer had any hair after chemotherapy? These decisions certainly added great meaning and comfort for us, as I know they could for many others.

The trips we took always were bittersweet. We relished the magnificent scenery of California, especially the national parks and the spectacular Pacific Coast. Erie continued to pursue her passion of taking hundreds of pictures on each trip, but she also knew that each experience likely was the last time she would see that place or share time with special friends and family members. She knew that she almost certainly would never enjoy her grandchildren. As she prepared to say goodbye to our sons, she hoped that they would both become fathers and pass on the love she felt. This denial of the opportunity to become a grandmother was especially difficult for her emotionally. She insisted on holding a joint engagement party for Nate and Dave and their fiancées, and Erie courageously and unexpectedly managed to stay alive long enough to see each of our boys get married. She surely would be thrilled to know that, within two years of her passing away, she did become a grandmother, in spirit, to both a grandson and a granddaughter, one on each coast.

Knowing that my life would continue without Erie for the first time after our 40 years together, I faced my own emotional challenges in trying to figure out how I wanted to live. Erie, always wise and grounded, encouraged me to seek out counseling before she died. And so, I did. This was not a comfortable ground for me. For 65 years, I had been accustomed to figuring out things on my own. I preferred it that way. I am not particularly self-reflective. I tend to approach each day, each situation, each problem, each opportunity on its own, without giving too much thought or concern to the long-term, big picture. To my surprise, I benefitted from her suggestion to seek professional guidance. I found an experienced psychologist whom I saw every few weeks for the last six months of Erie's life and continuing for several months thereafter. Each session gave me the opportunity to reflect on what was happening in our lives and, most importantly, what feelings and fears I was experiencing as Erie neared death. This is just another example of the positive impact that Erie had on those she loved. She knew that I tended to hold my emotions securely inside, and she knew that it would be much healthier for me to share those emotions in a safe, professional setting. Based on my experience, I would encourage others to seek counsel as part of their caregiver's role, even if the idea seems uncomfortable.

I had many practical concerns and emotional qualms about how I would continue life on my own. Did I want to stay in the house, surrounded by so many memories, happy and sad? Did I want to stay in the Sacramento area or relocate elsewhere? Did I have any interest in going back to work in any capacity, including working for a nonprofit entity, especially one involving environmental issues such as the protection of public lands and wildlife? What would I do with all of Erie's special possessions, including her thousands of wonderful photographs? Would I be interested in meeting someone else in due course, even though I knew that no one could replace Erie? From the counseling I received, and with the support of my sons, extended family, and dear friends, I realized that there was no need to rush into any of these decisions. The most important thing for me, in the immediate aftermath of Erie's death, was to take the time I needed to "process" my emotions following the loss of my best friend after 40 years. This idea of postponing big decisions soon after a death is generally well-known, yet it can be difficult to follow, as I occasionally discovered in the months and years after Erie died.

Before figuring out how best to give meaning to my own life, I felt a compelling need to spend more time creating the kind of legacy for Erie that my sons and I would cherish. I wrote an obituary for the local Sacramento Bee newspaper that attempted to capture not only the essential facts of her life, but also her warm and loving spirit and her wonderful, irascible sense of humor. I also planned a memorial service and celebration of life for our friends in the Sacramento community, along with family members, her doctors, and several close friends who traveled great distances to attend. This proved to be a wonderful, if bittersweet, way to express their feelings of love and appreciation for Erie. We held the service outdoors on April 22, 2017 - - Earth Day -- at the Women's Empowerment Program where she had worked for many years. We were blessed with a beautiful spring day and an abundance of heartfelt emotions and appreciation for the role that Erie had played in everyone's life.

While I generally try to be modest, I candidly take great pride and satisfaction in the way in which I cared for Erie during her extended illness, planned for her death, and celebrated her life. My experience as her caregiver proved to be the single most rewarding thing I have ever done and the event in my life for which I feel most proud today. In the end, I honestly felt like I did everything I possibly could to be a devoted husband, caregiver, and friend for the woman I loved. We were fortunate to have had 40 wonderful years together, to have raised two wonderful sons, and to have enjoyed our lives together, through good times and bad. And I will do everything possible to make sure that my sons and my young grandchildren appreciate the incredible warmth of spirit that Erie created during her life. Caring for her was an act of complete selflessness, devoting my time and efforts to the well-being of another human being for whom I cared deeply. I hope that others can take similar comfort in the caregiving roles that they provide.

Now, five years later, to bring some meaning to my life, and hers, I look each day at photos of Erie around the house. They are constant reminders of the wonderful years we spent together. I frequently go to "Erie's spot" along the American River in Sacramento where we often visited and picnicked with friends and family. I visit the Mendocino Botanical Gardens almost every year, where I have dedicated a plaque in her memory amidst the azalea gardens. The plaque reads: "In loving memory of Erie Arbisser Shockey. She loved these gardens and the magnificent ocean. May all who pass by here find peaceful tranquility." Next month, I will go to Mendocino again, this time with Nate, Felicia, Dave, Mandi, and my two three-year-old grandchildren. This will be the first time that all of us are united in a special place that Erie loved so much. I have spread her ashes along the American River and the Pacific Coast. On important dates, including her birthday, our wedding anniversary, and the annual "yahrzeit" marking the date of her death, I post a tribute to her on Facebook, along with several favorite pictures of Erie's smiling face. All these things help to remind me of her ongoing presence, even as I march ahead with my own life in her absence. One who has not personally lived with cancer can never truly know what it is like for the patient, living every day with a dreaded, terminal disease. How, I often ask myself, will I react when my time comes? I only hope that I am able to do so with some measure of the dignity and strength that was so apparent in both Erie and my mother. They were wonderful teachers and role models on how to live and how to die. Shalom. Peace.

# Paying it Forward

## By
## Cindy Bowden

We were living in a golf community that has two airstrips. One afternoon in the spring of 2019, I was standing at the kitchen sink and heard planes flying overhead. I found myself wondering if any of the neighborhood pilots would be willing to fly Randall to and from Houston if we would pay for their fuel. Randall drove himself to MD Anderson in the fall of 2018 and together, that winter we made trips weekly. Not only was he fighting for his life, but we were fighting traffic driving across the state and in Houston. Fighting stage 4 cancer is overwhelming and driving the 454 miles round trip increased the level of stress we experienced throughout the treatment journey. I called the pilot in charge of our airstrips and he told me about Angel Flights. John has no idea how much he improved our quality of life when he suggested that we contact them. Without the timely assistance of Angel Flights, Randall would not have been able to participate in clinical trials at MD Anderson. These amazing, generous pilots volunteer their time and planes to provide free air transportation for families in need. They provided over 70 free flights for Randall. After Randall's death, in lieu of flowers, I asked that donations be made to Angel Flights and Ground Angels. Ground Angels are people who volunteer their time and vehicles to drive patients from airports to their medical appointments. Our ground angel Sandra, even drove us to and from the radiation appointments those two weeks in March of 2021. She went above and beyond and I endeavor to pay it forward.

Our friend, pilot Rob, invited us to the Angel Flight Gala in February of 2020, where Randall was asked to speak after a retired Dallas Cowboy football player flown by Angel Flights and a female astronaut. I believe he opened with a remark about how humbling it was to follow such distinguished guest speakers—he was a little awed to be there. Toward the end of his speech, Randall said, "I work as a professor and department head for a university. I oversee 16 faculty, three master's programs, and one doctoral program. By helping me, Angel Flight reaches university faculty, hundreds and hundreds of students who are teachers, principals, and superintendents. By helping me, you serve college and university directors, deans, vice-presidents, and provosts. By helping me, you touch the lives of thousands of students from K-12 through higher education. By helping me, you impact colleagues, parents, and communities beyond measure." With a catch in his throat, Randall went on to say, "I really don't know how far-reaching Angel Flight generosity extends… But this I do know, I don't have the resources, and maybe not even the option to go to MD Anderson in Houston for world-class medical care, if it were not for Angel Flight South Central."

Tarleton State University was aware Randall was a cancer survivor when they recruited and hired him in the summer of 2018. Not only were we living in the right community at the right time for Randall to battle cancer at MDA in Houston; Randall was in the right position, at the right university when he was diagnosed with the stage 4 metastatic melanoma. Much like my principal, Randall's deans, Jordan and Kim endorsed every one of Randall's trips to MDA. After being in the Texas A&M system for years, Randall had accumulated hundreds of hours of sick time. The faculty and staff in the college of education at Tarleton State was extremely supportive of Randall. He worked full time at the university during his battle against cancer and took leave just nine days before he passed. Randall's colleagues in the educational leadership program at Tarleton State started the Dr. Randall Bowden Scholarship. The requirement for endowments is to have a minimum of $25,000 in place within 5 years. If it doesn't get to $25,000 within 5 years, it would be considered a funded scholarship, which would eventually deplete the funds. I cannot think of a more deserving university and community to benefit from the scholarship, nor can I think of a greater honor to bestow upon Randall, a man who served higher education for over 30 years. Up until his final days, Randall endeavored to ensure that his faculty and students deserved his best. I serve every day by teaching elementary school and aspire to live a meaningful life of service and exemplify the life of Randall, my OTH, who gave willingly of himself throughout his life.

# Evolving A Meaningful Life

## By
## Diane Linick

I am still sad and lost without David, but I now feel that I'm honoring David's life by sharing his wisdom about living a proud, and meaningful life. It's a wonderful way to remember David on a daily basis. I also get immense pleasure when I see how certain values are playing out in our children's and grandchildren's lives.

David lived an evolving meaningful life and adapted to changes by setting new goals for himself. David understood that your priorities sometimes also needed to be adjusted. At no time was that clearer than after David's cancer diagnosis. Obviously, cancer was our family's most difficult challenge. I knew David would do the best that he could to prolong his time doing what he felt defined him as a loving father and husband. I feel that through our many conversations during David's cancer journey he felt the need to show me his support of my ability to carry on the parental roles, something we both felt strongly about. This was an emotional issue for us to discuss. David's sharing his confidence in me meant a great deal going forward. I can't be David, but I'll always have his ideals combined with mine and like him, live by appreciating the beauty of each day and be there for family. Beginning in college and throughout our marriage there wasn't a day that David didn't acknowledge in some small way how he loved his life and never wasted a moment with trivial matters. What a beautiful legacy he left for our children and me.

For David there was no pretense to be other than who he was. Everyone David met was treated with respect and admiration. Friends and family, even strangers, knew they had David's full attention during any interaction. There was no surprise that David had been a sought after mentor to our children, nieces, and nephews. David was honored to be there for our next generation. You knew immediately David was listening to you, always in the present, thinking before he responded to your questions, and then offering his best advice which was always nonjudgmental. In fact, that was one of the reasons people wanted to be in his company, both socially and in business. David was known for his sense of humor and at the same time was considered trustworthy with private conversations and work matters. Like David, I prided myself on being a trusted spouse, parent, relative, friend, and teacher. I was really put to the test during David's cancer hurdles in his last few months. Friends and relatives were continually inquiring about how David was doing. Even though I knew that David trusted me to honor his need for normalcy and privacy, I did feel relief when he eventually voiced that he was ready to visit even with his extended family and friends. I learned from both my sister and my husband what determination to get the most out of your life looked like. I will always be in awe of how cancer patients display so much strength. ( I am in no way comparing a cancer patient or caregiver to the multitude of types of people offering care in totally different situations and for the vastly different lengths of time).

Over the years people have gone out of their way to let me know what a devoted and exceptional friend, coworker, and mentor David was to them and even to others in their families. David was modest about his acts of kindness because it was just how he lived his life. Most memorable to me about David was how, in so many aspects of his life, he became our family's role model of how to lead a good life. He exemplified a healthy lifestyle. His love of fresh air and exercise were expressed through golf, tennis, training, and running marathons and in local runs for various charities.

Nothing impresses me more than watching how our children have incorporated some of our qualities into their own lives. David's example of a life well lived was evident to many. We shared many of the same values and were happy to accept variations of each other's to be the best examples of loving parents and hardworking responsible adults.

Following David's cancer diagnosis, he fought hard to maintain a healthy lifestyle as he had created for himself years earlier. Most of David's priorities in life were still evident during his cancer journey. He was dedicated to his family, hard work, healthy diet, daily exercise, running, and doing projects within our house, and gardening. David enjoyed working and providing guidance and support for everyone in our family. He was a loving and involved father and a beloved husband.

As a family, we had cheered David on by attending many local charitable races. Never did we think that he had major goals with this new interest. David was a very disciplined and organized person and modeled how to make a plan for yourself when learning something new. He researched how to prepare to be a runner. This led him to study which foods and meal planning would pair best for a runner. He went around to local sports stores to check out shoes and athletic wear and tried different workouts to see which worked best for him. It was an education for the kids and me as well, though never David's intention. As he improved, he pushed himself to train for longer races and kept detailed records of his times and personal bests. We loved traveling to other states to watch him run several marathons. We were able to see what runners put themselves through to work toward ever-increasing goals. We followed David as he ran 6 marathons. I was again in awe of what we learned from David as to what a meaningful life could look like. He trained, ate properly, worked hard, and felt proud. I was so amazed when after he died that our kids, on their own, decided and planned personal training schedules and ran one of the local races together! That was never David's overall plan, but nothing could have meant more to him! It just shows how being around someone who exemplifies a quality life can mean to those around them.

Running didn't work for me, however, that's when I was inspired to become a walker. David was my silent coach in many aspects of life. He had a way of stretching our little evening walk around the block into a wonderful extended walk out of our neighborhood. Walking and gardening supported David's favorite ways to relax. During David's cancer journey I wanted to do the same for him. I tried to now be the one to encourage David to continue this routine when not going through treatments. I believed he would feel a sense of calm and normalcy " being himself" at the end of the day. As much as the exercise, David loved being outside taking care of our beautiful, serene backyard. I could tell how weak David was feeling as those walks tapered off. I tried to motivate him by saying how much I had always enjoyed, needed, and appreciated his encouragement. When the weather was good and gardening was too strenuous, I would set up breakfast or dinner on our patio table overlooking the yard. It was a good way for both of us to take in the fresh air, relax, and enjoy the flowers in our gardens. To watch your loved one slowly abandon their "feel good" routines was very difficult for me.

# Creating A Meaningful Lifestyle

## By

## Sonja McCaughey

My granddaughter was diagnosed with leukemia when she was nine years old. She was very active in gymnastics and was on a competitive team. She was also learning how to play the piano, but she did not like sitting up straight for the piano teacher. Nikita was a fast learner when it came to learning to read music and her notes. She was vivacious in learning everything her parents exposed her to. As an Army brat, Nikita experienced being a world traveler and all the different cultures that came with living in different places. She learned how to make friends quickly. She learned how to cope with moving and leaving her friends behind. She learned how big the world was every time she got to visit a new place. She beat cancer.

As odd as it sounds, she was blessed in getting leukemia at the young age that she did. Neurologically her nerves were still developing so she did not experience the levels of physical pain that most leukemia patients go through. She was able to have her spinal taps without anesthesia because she learned how to adapt to the situation and overcome her fears of what was about to happen. Nikita did not lose all of her hair during all of her treatments. I don't know if that was due to all the prayers that were said to allow her to continue to be a little girl or the tenaciousness of her mother in making sure that she ate appropriate food and was treating her hair to resist medications. However, the time came when her hair needed to be cut and Nikita decided on a style of hats that she wanted to wear. She had her favorite hats that she knew looked good with her clothes and others that kept her warm; she was quite the style girl! When it was time for her to move to an apartment next to the hospital, the sparkle in her eyes came back. She absolutely understood that she had a weakened immune system and the importance of not being around people who could contaminate her and make her sick. If she were to run a fever, she had to see her doctors immediately. Having her in an apartment allowed her to have some of her childhood back. We were allowed to stay with her, eat with her, and play with her. As long as she felt good, we took outings to places she would enjoy. I don't know exactly how the Make A Wish Foundation learned about Nikita. I do know that someone has to refer a child. Once they approached her parents, the foundation selected Nikita for her wish. She was able to go to Punta Cana in the Dominican Republic with her family. She was able to be a little girl again even though she had to wear a lot of sunscreen lotion to protect her skin from burning. The smile on her face while she got to play with her brother and walk on the beach with her dad. Levi was able to see his mom and spend time with her. This place will always remain a meaningful, special place for her.

When Nikita turned 10 years old her Florida family traveled to Maryland to celebrate this milestone birthday. It had been months since she saw her little brother and it was wonderful to see them catch up with each other. We celebrated her birthday by going to eat at restaurants that she enjoyed and to places that she loved to visit. However, Nikita had changed; we all had changed. The realization of her cancer became known to her and you could see it in her face. She was tired and became reserved in her actions. She did hurt. She got tired very quickly and she learned that the things that she used to do she could not do any longer. She would get bad headaches. Her daredevil attitude of conquering anything that she had before the cancer diagnosis she now struggled to achieve. She was concerned about the port that had been placed in her chest and was careful that it did not get bumped into as she engaged in her day-to-day activities as a 10-year-old girl. But Nikita learned to cope with the situation just as she learned the importance of wearing a mask for her safety (finding cute masks pre-Covid was not easy).

Nikita went into remission fairly quickly; however, the aggressiveness of her cancer kept her at the hospital longer. Each day away from that phone call for her to go home was not allowing her meaningful life to occur. Each day away from the day she was diagnosed and closer to remission was the prayer asking for her meaningful life to continue. Nikita is fifteen years old. She works about 5 hours a week at a local pizza restaurant after school and in between sports and band practice. She puts all her money into savings, and she lives her life as any teenager would live. She loves God. She stays in contact with the friends she made during her cancer journey. She is acutely aware of people and somewhat shy. Her meaningful life is that she has tomorrow. My meaningful life for her is to see her grow old. So far, she is doing pretty good. Her hair is almost to her waist, and she is taller than me. Her beautiful blue eyes are vibrant, and her smile is no longer tired. She is back on the honor roll and after a soccer injury, she is rethinking what her next sport to conquer will be. She will be driving soon, dating, and graduating high school. I don't know where she will go to college, but I would love for her to live with me just long enough for me to have more memories. I still fear her early twenties, but I am enjoying watching her mature to fulfill her meaning in life.

My life has become more meaningful because I know my granddaughter is doing great and she has her future in front of her. I don't know what her plans will end up being, but she has the option to have one. I continued with my education however I have more passion to work for those in need. While in policing, people were in need because they were in distress and needed police officers to help them with the situation. I became less tolerant of dealing with people when the only time I saw them they were the victim, or they were the suspect. It's unfortunate that the longer a person is a police officer they become more cynical. I have a meaningful life and I want to give back to those because I want to and I can. Life is short and kindness is easy.

# Saying Goodbye and Life After Death

## By

## Elizabeth Hapner

Hope gave us the ability to stay positive for most of Kyle's journey and more importantly, the peace of mind as his life was ending that permitted both of us to let him go on to his eternal life. That hope came from our faith, which is one aspect of his situation that we did discuss on multiple occasions. The closer Kyle came to the end, the greater importance this knowledge took on. While we started with the hope that his condition would be operable, then that his treatment would be successful in greatly extending his life, we went on to hoping his transition to his afterlife would be peaceful. Days before his passing, having come to a point of acceptance and peace, Kyle expressed his concern about me once he was gone and I told him that when he was ready to go, it was okay to let go of the pain. Making certain that he knew I would miss him constantly for the rest of my life, I was equally determined that he would understand that I would be at peace also because I knew that he would be relieved of his pain, enjoying Paradise, and looking forward to the day when we would be reunited.

Saying goodbye to a loved one, and most especially your child, is the most difficult thing we do in life. How do you say goodbye to the center of your universe? Relying on my God is the only way I have been able to negotiate this unnatural situation. I had always teased Kyle that pay backs are hell and he was going to remember that when he had to look after me in my old age. No one expects to bury their child. Without my faith to sustain me, I cannot imagine how I would have survived this incredible loss.

We went through several periods where we were told Kyle's death was imminent. Each time, Kyle defied the odds through sheer persistence. Simply put, he was not ready to leave us. On Kyle's thirty-second birthday, March 24, 2020, he was clearly waning. Friends brought him an ice cream cake and gifts but he could not get up and was not feeling sociable, so their visit was short-lived. Three days later, he was in such pain and unable to take in any nutrition that I arranged for him to go to Moffitt Urgent Care by ambulance. Travel by car was just too difficult for him by this juncture.

Already into the pandemic, the entire Moffitt facility was on lockdown. Thankfully, I was permitted to stay with Kyle as long as I did not leave the room. Lack of food, shower, and change of clothes was a small sacrifice under the circumstances. Approximately twelve hours later, shortly after midnight, he was admitted to a room and I was permitted to go with him and get him settled before I had to leave. A tube was to be inserted into his colon later that day. Leaving him alone at that point was incredibly difficult because there was no assurance that he would be returning home.

So early in the pandemic, staff had not really adapted to the idea of updating family by phone. Obtaining information was difficult and Kyle was not feeling up to much communication himself. Later, Kyle told me that staff had said, within his earshot, that he would not likely survive and return home. Determined that this would not be the case, Kyle simply used force of will to return home to us. Again, because of the pandemic, I was not given any training or real information as to what to expect with this tube and stoma. Kyle's supportive care physician saw him in the hospital, prescribing his IV pain pump and offering him emotional support in my absence.

Kyle was sent home with Hospice which had benefits and drawbacks. Hospice care permitted him to come home with a Morphine pain pump which made his pain level somewhat more manageable. At the same time, we had Hospice workers with us twenty-four/seven which Kyle found uncomfortable. Generally speaking, there was not much for them to do so when he was deemed "stable" after five days, they switched to weekly visits by the nurse and changes to his pain medication bags, as needed. While Kyle preferred this, it was very difficult to move him to change the dressings and bathe him. It also left me in the position of figuring out care of the stoma on my own. Thankfully, a friend from high school had been through this with her late husband months earlier and she was invaluable to me, educating me on which supplies were best and how to clean around the stoma.

Stomas take approximately eight weeks to heal so Kyle's was always raw. The supplies provided by Moffitt and by Hospice were not the best ones for Kyle. My friend gave me some supplies she had left and told me where to order more. Because Kyle's pain level never dropped below an 8, with the tube, Hospice wanted to admit him to a Hospice house. Kyle refused, wanting the comfort of home and fewer restrictions in seeing people. As he said, his pain level had never been as low as they felt they could get it at Hospice House, even when he was in the hospital, so he saw no point in otherwise sacrificing his comfort in an effort to lower his pain level. Candidly, he felt Hospice would quicken his demise by increasing his pain medication.

One of Kyle's primary concerns, understandably, was what dying would actually be like. During his last physical visit to Moffitt, several months prior to his death, he asked his oncologist whether he would be gasping for breath, in more severe pain or just how death would come. His oncologist assured him that he would just go to sleep and not awaken again, which eased his mind tremendously. This is exactly what occurred.

Kyle's supportive care physician, another wonderful healthcare provider, discussed with Kyle, during our last office visit with her, the concept of "fighting" cancer and the "war on cancer." Suggesting that we should not view it in that fashion but look at it as a part of life's natural course and the segue way to Heaven. While we understood her point that it could be negative energy, neither of us viewed it that way nor were ready to concede the "fight." Kyle had fought too long and too hard to stay with us longer and had not reached the point that he was ready to let go.

Curious about the origin of the origin of the "war on cancer." I researched it and learned it became part of our culture when President Nixon declared the "war on cancer" after it became the second leading cause of death in our country.

To this day, I struggle with the fact that while there were 16.9 million cancer survivors as of 1999, and cancer is now generally a treatable illness, my Kyle was not one of the fortunate ones. Given his young age and good health otherwise, accepting his terminal diagnosis was incredibly hard then and still is. My only solace is my belief that he is in a better place, with nothing but happiness. A client who lost his twin brother to stomach cancer, and who has had several near death experiences, told me that he now has no doubt whatsoever that his brother, my son, and others are in Paradise. Neither of us has any fear of dying.

Hospice is a wonderful organization and we certainly benefitted overall from their services, but Kyle's situation differed from many. Available service was limited, especially so early in the pandemic when staff was quite low. When we first consulted with Hospice, they did not think Kyle was ready for their services. By the time we received their services, there was not a lot for Hospice to do, aside from pain management.

Pain management by morphine pump was invaluable to Kyle but not without its challenges. Several times Kyle was left without morphine in his pain pump and had to take oral medication on a temporary basis. Oral medication was not as effective, and he was left in severe pain for hours each time while the problems were rectified. On one occasion, the Hospice worker did not properly attach the pump and it leaked all over the floor, leaving Kyle without liquid medication until they could get another ordered and delivered. On a couple of other occasions, the Hospice workers did not get there in time to install the new medication bag before his prior one was empty.

Although Kyle was confident that he was going to a place with no pain, where he would be reunited with his friend, Matt, and others who had preceded him, it was still difficult to say goodbye to his earthly friends, family and his beloved Kylie. In the last weeks, he could not tolerate having anyone on his bed so Kylie could not go in his room unless someone was with her to keep her off his bed. Pandemic measures restricted visitors so Kyle said the majority of his goodbyes by Facetime or phone. Even news of his death was primarily by Facebook because of the pandemic. Despite my decision to delay his memorial service for a year to allow pandemic measures to abate, the pandemic was still in effect, and limited attendance. Two of his closest friends ended up with COVID at the time of his service and had to watch it on YouTube.

Having no idea when Kyle's passing would occur, he and I had said our goodbyes in various fashion, a number of times over his last few weeks. On his last day on Earth, he had developed bedsores along his spine. Although this was an indication that he did not have much time left, I did not anticipate that his death was coming as soon as it did. A close friend of Kyle's had been by daily, assisting me with attending to his physical requirements. While I went to the pharmacy to buy bandaging for his bedsores, Kyle took him that he was ready to go but was concerned about me.

Unaware of Kyle's statement until after his death, I did not expect him to leave me for another day or two. Once he came to the decision that he was ready, it was just a matter of hours. Several times that night, he asked me to push the button on his pain pump for him. Until 3:30 a.m. that morning, I was with Kyle, pressing his pain pump every fifteen minutes. After that, he fell asleep and I went to bed, fully believing that I would see him in the morning. Sometime in that couple of hours, he passed away. While I would have preferred to be there when he passed, I feel confident that he did not awaken again. We had prepared for this moment over the prior several weeks, never knowing when it would be the final goodbye.

Having Hospice made the details of his passing much easier, and I would highly recommend that to anyone. Our preference as to funeral home was already made known to them. No emergency rescue or law enforcement was called as it was considered an attended death and the Hospice doctor signed the death certificate. Our Hospice nurse took care of removing their equipment and the soiled bedding. I simply said my post passing goodbyes and bagged all the unused medication for Hospice to take. I was otherwise free to spend my time with the close friends who came over to support me. Hospice also offers free grief counseling and followed up several times to make certain I was aware of the availability of those services.

The courage and unwavering faith Kyle displayed throughout his illness continue to inspire me. The gratitude he never failed to express to all the caregivers, and to me, made me consistently proud as well. Initially, the idea of saying goodbye was absolutely incomprehensible. Watching Kyle in such pain during his final weeks made me realize that this was just selfish. As his parent and the person closest to him, it was my job to make it easier for him to make that transition to eternal life when the time came.

The reality of eventual death has caused me to give more consideration to planning. As an attorney, I have my estate plan in place. As a single female with no living offspring or parents, I have had to make more detailed efforts to ensure that no one will be unduly burdened with the responsibility of handling my estate affairs. I have yet to undertake letters to leave for my close friends but have made lists of people who need to be contacted. Physically, I chose to have his ashes buried with those of my parents and brother in our church memory garden and my ashes will someday join them.

In the course of my law practice, and life in general, I have seen far too many instances in which a loved one was suddenly gone, without warning. Personally, that has been the situation with every death I have experienced in my immediate family prior to Kyle's. The opportunity to let your child (or other loved one) know just how precious he is to you and how grateful you are for the time together, and to say goodbye, is such a precious gift. Every time I start to think of all the milestones Kyle missed out on and all the things we will never have the opportunity to share, such as another generation,

I just remember all the opportunities I had to let him know how much I loved him and looked forward to being reunited someday. As I tell all my estate planning clients, tomorrow is not guaranteed so plan accordingly.

Kyle's death has caused me to live more meaningfully. While I have always dedicated many hours to pro bono work and community service, I have experienced a new dedication to that work in his memory. It has also given me a new perspective in dealing with clients' emotional needs. Kindness is something I always try to offer all, knowing that I generally have no idea what is going on in their lives. My goal is to improve at least one person's life each day and to leave the world a better place when I am reunited with Kyle and other loved ones.

The legacy of love and memories Kyle left is my treasure now. The process of going from pure grief over a photo or memory to finding comfort in those same things takes a while but my faith allowed me to reach that turning point much earlier than I would have anticipated. I do not hesitate to say "Kyle loved this" or "Kyle and I did that" when a topic comes up. Tears still come occasionally as I will always miss him tremendously but primarily, I am grateful for the blessing of more than thirty-two years of life and love shared with him.

# Epilogue

# Lessons Learned

"You have cancer." Three terrifying words for a cancer patient and for the cancer caregiver. Hearing those words turns their world upside down and creates a sense of chaos for the patient and their family as they come to terms with the "new normal" as they determine how to battle cancer while trying to lead a regular life doing the things they used to do before receiving a cancer diagnosis.

Our writers have shared with us that their journeys alongside their loved ones often mirrored the patients' journeys. The caregivers initially found themselves at a loss to know exactly what to do and they often struggled to balance their own life while meeting the needs of their loved ones. As noted by more than one of our writers, each caregiver's journey is different. They searched for the best ways to help their loved ones while trying to respect the needs and wishes of their loved ones. The fundamental questions asked were: "How can I best help and what is my role in this battle?"

The best strategies to provide the optimum care and help for the cancer traveler are not always evident at the outset of the journey. It takes time to determine what will work best for the individual caregiver in his/her particular situation. What works for one cancer patient does not necessarily work for another in the same way. It takes time to discern the appropriate approach for each caregiver's "routine" to help their loved ones who have been thrust into the most difficult struggles of their lives. It is an "uncomfortable reality" for everyone involved in the cancer journey. As all cancer travelers and caregivers have learned, life is not fair and it is not an easy process. No day was the same for our caregivers and they each had to take time to notice what the cancer patient was experiencing and to learn the most appropriate and effective actions to take so they did not make a bad day worse for the patient.

Our caregiver travelers were working in their chosen professions at the time they made the transition to a cancer caregiver after their loved one's diagnosis of cancer. They each reacted with shock and fear when they learned of the cancer diagnosis. At the time of their entry into the role of caregiver, most of the writers had not experienced significant exposure to cancer. Some had said goodbye to parents and grandparents but had not been in a "direct" caregiver's role. Each caregiver dealt with the difficulty of helping the patient retain their "pre-cancer" identity so they would not be known simply as a cancer patient. Each worked hard to establish a routine to allow the patient to be "their own person" while at the same time being present for the patient so they could depend on them.

One concept that was a major concern for each of our caregivers was that of time. It is the great unknown that came with the cancer diagnosis, not just in terms of how much time they would have with their loved one, but also in other ways.

One obvious first step taken by each of the caregivers was to spend time learning as much as they could about the type of cancer they and their loved ones were dealing with. After processing the shock and the related emotions that came with the devastating news of the cancer diagnosis, each caregiver searched for information and struggled to absorb as much of the information provided by the medical teams as possible. They were inquisitive, demanding and persistent, asking many questions during their searches for the most current and complete information about cancer so they could fully understand the complicated processes necessary to treat cancer so they could provide "outside" counsel for their loved ones and they could serve as another set of eyes and ears and be a "thoughtful patient advocate" as Diane Linick stated.

Charlie and Erie immersed themselves in finding out as much as they could about breast cancer and the best treatment options available at the time of her original diagnosis. Linda and Diane each became the notetaker for their husbands during the seemingly endless meetings with the medical teams who provided treatment for the cancers. Diane would carefully read her notes to her husband so he could fully understand his cancer and the difficult processes they would be facing to treat the metastatic melanoma. Linda shared her notes from the meetings with the medical team at Moffitt Cancer Center with her husband Dave and also discussed his health status during her "roundtable" sessions with friends from church. The notes became a journal of the reluctant journey into the battle against cancer.

Cindy bird-dogged the staff at M.D. Anderson to make sure they reviewed Randall's charts and made the correct diagnosis for Randall's cancer to set up the correct strategy for beating the germ cell cancer. This process was repeated two years later when Randall was diagnosed with metastatic melanoma. Cindy briefly stepped away from teaching and became the "travel coordinator" to allow Randall, to travel to M.D. Anderson for treatments without having to endure the long hours on the road driving to Houston from Corpus Christi and later from Granbury to Houston. The burden of planning the visits to M.D. Anderson became much easier when Angel Flight provided flights to and from Houston as Randall battled the cancer. They were a "godsend" to her and Randall in their battle.

Skyp wanted to learn as much as she could about Nikita's fall, but she faced the difficult logistics of trying to provide support from Florida while Nikita and her parents were at Walter Reed Medical Center in Washington. Skyp later provided support and care for her grandson while trying to be a strong presence to help her granddaughter during the early stages of her cancer treatments. As a result of being thrust into the role of caregiver, Skyp moved up her retirement from the Tampa Police Department so she could be present for her son's family as they transitioned from his duty station in Germany back to the United States.

How much time do we have left? Each of our caregivers dealt with that issue in different ways, depending on the type of cancer and the prognosis provided by the medical care providers. As our caregivers have shown, cancer is generally a prolonged illness and does not care what physical condition the patient is in when they are diagnosed. They can be in good physical condition, as Randall Bowden and David Linick were both avid runners and had competed in marathons and triathlons. Kyle Rockhill was a fit 30-year old man who did not fit the profile for colon cancer. Skyp's granddaughter Nikita was a typical, active and healthy 9-year old when she received her diagnosis. Erie

Shockey and Dave Devine, while having been smokers in the past, were in relatively good health at the time of their respective diagnoses.

After Erie's breast cancer went into remission, Charlie and Erie were blessed to have 20 years before the cancer returned. They relocated from the Washington, D.C. area to Sacramento and Charlie continued his career with DOJ until he retired to devote his time to Erie's needs after her cancer returned. The gift of time allowed them to travel to Israel for their sons' bar mitzvahs ceremonies and take other family trips before the cancer's return. They visited national parks and traveled to Houston in their "Silver Lining" convertible and maximized their remaining time together.

Linda and Dave Devine were fortunate as Dave beat the lung cancer diagnosis and he came through the removal of a malignant brain tumor with no serious side effects. These milestones provided more time together but caused a major shift in Linda's life. Linda had a strong support group from her colleagues at the university and from the "First Reformed Prayer Chain" from her church and her roundtable friends. She and Dave had numerous roundtable sessions to discuss and process what they were experiencing. Dave is a "glass half full" person and they both believed they had better odds with the cancer with that approach. But, as Linda noted, what was had been lost and it would be no more, even though she and Dave are fortunate enough to have more time together. Diane and David Linick worked hard to balance their time together. David wanted to retain his "non-cancer" identity and to continue contributing to his legal career, his family and other favorite pastimes. David continued his work as an attorney and was fortunate to be able to handle much of his caseload from home. While David's running days were behind him, he was able to continue gardening in his backyard and taking walks with Diane in the neighborhood. Diane treasured every opportunity to be with David during his cancer battle.

Cindy's time was also precious as Randall's condition necessitated frequent trips and hospital stays at M.D. Anderson for his treatments. Randall managed to continue working at the universities throughout his treatments although his physical condition worsened. She and Randall took time to reflect on their good fortune that they lived in Texas, and they were able to avail themselves of the tremendous resources at M.D. Anderson Hospital in Houston. They beat cancer once, but it came back with a vengeance.

Skyp was fortunate that she got to have quality time with her granddaughter while she was in the early treatment stages. She also has received the gift of time as Nikita's cancer has gone into remission and she has time to watch her granddaughter grow up and spend time with her grandson to get to know him better. She learned to balance family time with other responsibilities.

Betsey was able to provide ongoing and consistent support for Kyle during his illness and they were able to spend quality time together in his final months. As they struggled to navigate the often confusing pathways of the health care system to get Kyle the best care possible, the onset of the pandemic provided more time for them as the court system shut down and switched to virtual hearings. Betsey used that gift of more time together to balance her emotions so she would have the strength to meet and support Kyle's needs on his cancer journey.

As our caregivers traveled on their reluctant journey, they needed time to pause and reflect on their current situations and their priorities. Caring for their loved ones was most important and it was often necessary to change their routines to help meet the needs of the cancer patient. However, they each found it critically important to take care of themselves as well. It is easy to get caught up in the cancer patient's journey and overlook or forget about their own needs. As our caregivers noted, it is necessary to take care of their own needs or they may find that they have made the cancer patient's day worse. In so doing, don't be hesitant to accept offers of support from friends and colleagues. They are well-meaning and want to help during time of critical and significant difficulties. Take the time to realize you cannot do it all and that it is okay to accept offers of help during this stressful time in your life.

It is important to realize that the journey is taking a toll on the caregiver, and they must find the most appropriate way to cope with the stress of the journey. Whether it is a "roundtable" session at a local restaurant, going out with colleagues from work, or simply taking time to enjoy a meal with others can be a huge boost in the caregiver's morale and well-being. Finding a time to "decompress" after a long day can be extremely helpful in finding meaning in the everyday and in finding a sense of peace, if only for a short while. As Betsey noted, it is extremely important to be well rested during the journey. It is a difficult and often devastating time for the caregiver, and getting adequate rest is a must!

Another aspect of time for the caregiver is preparing for the end if the cancer patient's condition is terminal. It is important to include the family in conversations about the cancer patient's condition and situation and to fully express your feelings before the end comes and to address any other concerns. The caregiver must be patient and not rush or hide their true feelings. Take whatever time is needed to share your thoughts and emotions and to reflect on the life of the cancer patient. Each of our caregivers found the most appropriate way to do that during their respective journey. Diane and David shared precious time together on their walks in the neighborhood and in their garden, finding meaning in the everyday. Betsey and Kyle had wonderful, but difficult conversations over the course of Kyle's treatments up to the time of his passing. Charlie and Erie spent hours together before and during their "Silver Convertible" trips discussing what needed to be done at the end of her life. Cindy and Randall spent quality time together in similar conversations. While Linda and Skyp found themselves in different situations, they likewise used their time with their families to discuss and prepare for whatever unforeseen circumstances came their way as their loved ones went through their treatments

Regardless of our caregivers' religious beliefs, they showed it is vitally important to rely on faith to help guide them through the difficult challenges that come with the cancer diagnosis. Their faith helped them as they made their way through the often confusing and scary world of cancer and cancer treatment and in dealing with the loss of their loved ones. They have showed us how faith has helped them through difficult periods of uncertainty and mourning and ultimately how faith has helped them to find meaning in the loss of a loved one and how it has helped to show them a path from anguish and grief to a path of comfort toward a meaningful life.

We know the caregivers have struggled at times to share their stories for this book and we thank them for their time and contributions to this effort.

David Persky, Ph.D., J.D.

Got an idea for a book? Contact Curry Brothers Publishing, LLC. We are not satisfied until your publishing dreams come true. We specialize in all genres of books, especially religion, self-help, leadership, family history, poetry, and children's literature. There is an African Proverb that confirms, *"When an elder dies, a library closes."* Be careful who tells your family history. Our staff will navigate you through the entire publishing process, and we take pride in going the extra mile in meeting your publishing goals. Improving the world one book at a time!

Curry Brothers Publishing, LLC PO Box 247 Haymarket, VA 20168 (719) 466-7518 & (615) 347-9124

Visit us at: http://www.currybrotherspublishing.com

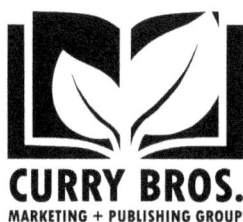

**CURRY BROS.**
MARKETING + PUBLISHING GROUP

www.ingramcontent.com/pod-product-compliance
Lightning Source LLC
Chambersburg PA
CBHW052111030426
42335CB00025B/2942